Stop Carrying *the Weight* of Your MS

Advance Praise

"Andrea Hanson offers practical, no-nonsense, yet compassionate solutions to help people with MS maximize their health. She starts by inviting the reader to join their healthcare team as the leader, to figuratively get into the driver's seat as the one person who knows intuitively what's best for them. She empowers the reader's inner change agent to visualize the future they want to live. Throughout *Stop Carrying the Weight of Your MS*, Andrea's friendly voice offers practical strategies for developing healthy behaviors towards eating and exercising: a particularly challenging problem for people with chronic health conditions like MS. Andrea seamlessly incorporates self-reflective questions and exemplar case studies to guide the reader in developing positive health behaviors which, in turn, help the reader visualize their long term weight and health goals. Thank you, Andrea!"

— **Janet Morrison** RN, MSN, MSCN,
The University of Texas at Austin, School of Nursing
Doctoral Candidate, ACE Certified Personal Trainer,
ACSM/NCHPAD Certified Inclusive Fitness Trainer

"Absolutely everyone who wants to lose weight should read this book. Knowing ahead of time how to stay consistent and not burn out is crucial to your success, especially when you have a chronic illness. I watch people in my gym start out strong in their workouts and then about 80% of them drop out and return to the couch. The cycle of stopping and starting diets, gaining and losing weight, is very stressful on your body. It negatively affects you on a systemic basis. Physiologically it stresses the hormonal system to a high degree and there can be nutrient loss through changes that are too aggressive too soon. The muscles, metabolism, and stamina of the body return to where it was before working out, leaving that person frustrated and unmotivated to try again. Some people will maintain better than others, but a majority of people will lose it all and then some. Having a plan like Andrea's that helps to solve the problem of stopping and starting is essential for weight loss. The most important thing for your body is to be consistent with diet and exercise and this is by far the best book I've read that helps with that. I will definitely share this book with clients who are having a hard time sticking with the changes needed to lose weight. Exercise is vital for your body's health, but understanding how to get your mind in the game and how your body reacts to your workouts are also essential parts of getting fit. Andrea Hanson's book effortlessly teaches this and more."

– **Kurt Pitman**, C.H.E.K Practitioner,
Olympic Lifting Coach, NMT, Metabolic Typing Advisor

Stop
Carrying
the Weight
of Your MS

The Art of *Losing Weight,*
Healing Your Body, and
Soothing Your Multiple Sclerosis

Andrea Wildenthal Hanson

NEW YORK

NASHVILLE • MELBOURNE • VANCOUVER

Stop Carrying *the Weight* of Your MS
The Art of *Losing Weight, Healing* Your Body, and *Soothing* Your Multiple Sclerosis

Published in New York, New York, by Morgan James Publishing. Morgan James and The Entrepreneurial Publisher are trademarks of Morgan James, LLC. www.MorganJamesPublishing.com

The Morgan James Speakers Group can bring authors to your live event. For more information or to book an event visit The Morgan James Speakers Group at www.TheMorganJamesSpeakersGroup.com.

Shelfie

A **free** eBook edition is available with the purchase of this print book.

CLEARLY PRINT YOUR NAME ABOVE IN UPPER CASE

Instructions to claim your free eBook edition:
1. Download the Shelfie app for Android or iOS
2. Write your name in **UPPER CASE** above
3. Use the Shelfie app to submit a photo
4. Download your eBook to any device

ISBN 978-1-68350-198-5 paperback
ISBN 978-1-68350-200-5 eBook
ISBN 978-1-68350-199-2 hardcover
Library of Congress Control Number:
2016914026

Cover Design by:
Rachel Lopez
www.r2cdesign.com

Editing:
Grace Kerina

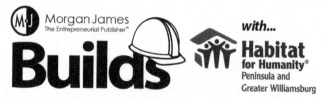

In an effort to support local communities, raise awareness and funds, Morgan James Publishing donates a percentage of all book sales for the life of each book to Habitat for Humanity Peninsula and Greater Williamsburg.

Get involved today! Visit
www.MorganJamesBuilds.com

DISCLAIMER

Neither the author nor the publisher assumes any responsibility for errors, omissions, or contrary interpretations of the subject matter herein. Any perceived slight of any individual or organization is purely unintentional.

Confidentiality is taken seriously and all names and identifying information in case studies and client stories have been changed. Stories shared about the author's experiences are detailed from her memories and her perspective only. Any resemblance, within this book, to real persons living or dead is purely coincidental apart from the author's own stories that are true to her.

This book contains discussions about health issues and medical problems. By reading this book, you acknowledge that the author is not a licensed psychologist, physician or other health care professional and the author's opinions in this book do not replace the care of psychologists, physicians or other healthcare professionals. If you have questions about a medical problem, please refer to you your physician, psychologist or other healthcare professional. The author's opinions in this book in no way are to be construed as or substituted for medical advice, psychological counseling, or any other type of therapy. The author cannot guarantee the outcome of coaching efforts and/or recommendations in this book and the author's comments about the outcome are expressions of her opinion only. In addition, please be advised that the author cannot be held responsible for medical decisions that you make as a result of reading this book. Please consult your physician or healthcare professional before making any changes in your health habits or diet.

Dedication

Here's to seeing results, instead of struggles.
To being your own hero, instead of waiting
for a knight in shining armor.
To understanding the key,
instead of only hoping for answers.
To knowing in your bones that this will work,
instead of wondering what to do and being stuck.

My teachers helped me see this
way of living as a reality.
This book is written with the support
of their wisdom, generosity, and love,
so that you may you see this way of
living as a reality, too.

Table of Contents

Foreword

For almost thirty years my colleagues and I have conducted multiple research studies focusing on the impact of a healthy lifestyle for persons with MS. When we first began this work, long before there were books or websites about wellness and MS (yes, even before there was an internet), our participants told us "We can get the general health message everywhere and we can get messages about our MS – but how do we put those together in a way that works for our individual lives?" This book by Andrea Hanson, *Stop Carrying the Weight of Your MS*, answers that often asked and rarely answered question.

Ms. Hanson provides essential tools and strategies that are useful for achieving a healthy weight and enhancing overall health while living with MS. Throughout this well-written book Ms. Hanson skillfully weaves in her own journey to a healthier lifestyle and the experiences of clients in her coaching business to help illustrate how change can actually happen. She highlights the importance of individual choice in determining what is the healthiest choice in the context of one's life. She then empowers individuals to move forward using a process and specific strategies, including achieving self-awareness, embracing self-management, and, most importantly, finding motivation.

My colleagues and I were among the very first researchers to study what persons with MS could do to improve their *health*. In contrast to most researchers who focused on the losses and symptoms of MS, we focused on what individuals with MS could do for themselves to enhance their overall health and quality of life. Over the years, more than 1,500 persons with MS have shared not only the data we requested from them, but also their stories, their lives, what worked and what didn't work. We have listened, knowing – as Ms. Hanson reminds readers here – that each individual is the expert on his/her own health and should be sitting at the "head of the table." We know that better quality of life and better outcomes are consistent with self-management. The messages imbedded in this book are consistent with what we have learned from many persons with MS, and with the strategies that we have tested and found effective in our clinical trials to improve health behaviors (physical activity, healthy eating, stress management), overall health, and quality of life.

As most readers know, MS is a chronic condition – meaning that individuals will live with it and its effects for many years. Ms. Hanson reminds readers that while having MS does not define your health, it does interact with your health. This means that you can be more or less healthy while living your life with this condition. Ms. Hanson provides tools to help readers decide how to live their life in as healthy a way as they may choose, emphasizing the importance of awareness, listening to your body, focusing on overall lifestyle, and motivation to change.

Our research confirms the logical idea that if you take steps to support your overall health – you exercise to maintain mobility, strength, and flexibility; you eat well to maintain energy and a healthy weight; and you manage stress and emotions in positive ways – you will have a better quality of life. While there will clearly be ups and downs in your ability to maintain a healthy lifestyle – our longitudinal research over a 20-year time period demonstrates that those with a healthier lifestyle develop fewer limitations related to their MS. We do not know if this is because healthy behaviors influence the disease process in some way or – perhaps what is more likely – those who engage in these behaviors are in better shape to withstand whatever life may bring them.

An important key message throughout this book is the idea of the individual as the expert on his or her own health. As the expert, sitting at the head of the table, you can use information provided by others to design what works best for you. With regard to exercise, Hanson states: "You can do anything you like for exercise. As long as your body is moving and you're exerting energy, you're good. Playing with your kids, going out on the water with the kayak club, or going for a walk are all great things to do. And there are many more options. It doesn't matter what you do as long as you do something."

That passage reminds me of a very special woman I met in one of my research projects over 20 years ago. She had come to her appointment at the School of Nursing and I met her at the front door of the building. She was clearly very "fit" and literally radiated good health – despite her significant difficulty walking, largely due to spasticity in her legs. We walked the distance to my research office while she held on to my upper arm with a tight grip. As we sat down and began the interview, I asked her what kinds of things she did to promote her health. She said, "Oh, I exercise every day." I asked her to tell me more about that and was somewhat stunned when she said, "I roller skate for about an hour several times a week." Given the great difficulty she had with walking, I could not imagine she would have the balance and strength required to roller skate. I asked her how she managed to do it and she responded, "Well – I was watching my kids roller skate with the neighbors and they were laughing and having so much fun. So I sent my husband to the store to buy me some skates. I told him to get the kind that lace up – no Velcro for me – that way I could work on my fine motor coordination too. Then I had him put a good sturdy lawn chair in the garage with a fan nearby to keep me cool. And I managed to get those skates on, sit in the chair and move by legs back and forth 'skating' while watching the kids laughing and playing. When I start to get tired, I scrunch down in the chair so that I'm working my thighs and not just my calves."

I learned several important things that day that I have never forgotten – most importantly the ability of individuals to adapt a "fun" activity that they wanted to do. And – because it's fun and pleasant to them – they do it. The results were evident – this woman had a healthy weight, a positive frame of mind from accomplishing what she wanted, good relationships with children and others, and leg muscles strong enough to help her maintain her balance and mobility in the face of some very challenging MS symptoms.

Ms. Hanson's observations and recommendations are consistent with a wide range of research – including our own with persons with MS – identifying useful approaches to improve health behaviors. She highlights the importance of identifying sources of support and potential barriers or roadblocks to change, and the powerful impact of believing in your ability to accomplish a goal. Indeed, the single greatest predictor of a wide range of behaviors, including eating healthy and exercising, is the person's own belief and confidence that he/she can accomplish the behavior, and the expectancy that it will have a positive outcome. Think of how many people – with or without MS – who accomplish something that makes you think, "She should never have been able to do that! She wasn't strong enough, bright enough or talented enough – but she did it!" You can bet that each of those successes occurred in the context of the individual's strong, unwavering belief that he/she would be successful and would accomplish the goal. Over and over, in all kinds of contexts, researchers have demonstrated that beliefs are stronger predictors than actual abilities.

In conclusion, I've learned many lessons in my thirty years of research focusing on the role of a healthy lifestyle to improve quality of life for persons with MS. This book is consistent with scientific "evidence" regarding individual change, and provides the essential and much needed "next step" – the tools and process that each person who reads this text can use in their own life. Every day brings a chance to get healthier and with this book you will have resources to help you on that journey.

Alexa Stuifbergen, PhD, RN, FAAN

Dean

James Dougherty Centennial Professor of Nursing

The University of Texas at Austin

Chapter 1

Important Questions

Abby was diagnosed with multiple sclerosis five years ago. Like many people facing a diagnosis, she was shocked when she heard the news. In her eyes, too much testing and time went by before she got the diagnosis. But at least, finally, she had an answer to what was happening to her.

Before her diagnosis, her legs kept tingling and feeling like pins and needles. She went to the doctor each time it happened, but was told that being overweight was most likely compressing a nerve in her back. The pins and needles would go away periodically, and so she thought she was fine.

Until she wasn't.

Now she has an explanation for what's going on with her health and has done her research on MS. She's lucky to have a good neurologist and drug treatment options. She knows – for the most part – what's happening with her body. She also knows that there's a lot she can do on her own to help her prognosis with this disease.

Abby is smart and can be categorized as an overachiever, although she just sees it as getting stuff done. She's the go-to for everything at her job and in her family. She likes it that way. Even though sometimes she wishes people would figure it out themselves, she's glad to be the "fixer."

Abby is doing well at work and sees promotion in her future. In fact, she sees a lot in her future – family, travel, adventures. What she never saw in her future was disability, illness, and hospital bills. When she's being totally honest with herself, a future involving any kind of dependency scares the hell out of her. *What if MS wrecks my life?*

Right now, she's doing well enough. The pins and needles in her legs are still there, but she can handle that. Other symptoms, like optic neuritis, have come and gone, but she gets steroids each time and recovers. She's strong, and she relies on that strength every day. But she can't help wondering, *if I'm so strong that I can have this great career, support my family and go out with friends, then why am I not strong enough to lose this extra weight?*

She tells herself that she should have this weight thing figured out by now.

It has occurred to her that she might have been accurately diagnosed with MS years earlier if she had been at a healthier body weight. *If the doctor didn't have weight to blame, would he have considered testing for MS sooner?* That's a question she knows will never be answered. But her motive still stands: if she wants to have that future without being dependent on someone else, she knows she needs to be as healthy as possible, starting now.

And she knows that means losing weight.

She was overweight before her diagnosis, so this isn't a new issue for her. But since then she's put on even more weight. Some of the weight is definitely from the steroids. *Those things are evil,* she tells herself. But she knows the steroids aren't the only things to blame for her weight. There isn't good food at the office, and her husband keeps junk food well-stocked in the kitchen at home. She feels sabotaged every time she turns around, and then there's the added pressure of MS on top of it.

I have to get on top of this, she tells herself.

Now that MS is in play, Abby is even more motivated to lose weight – and to do it the "right" way. She wants to exercise, but she doesn't love her options. She knows she wants to clean up her diet, but is unclear on the best things to eat (and not eat) for a person who has MS. She doesn't want to simply jump into something, and she knows she can lose weight and help her MS at the same time – *but how?*

She gets online to try and figure it out. There is no shortage of direct instructions in her research. She finds countless nutritionists, dieticians, doctors, and naturopaths that tell her exactly what to eat and what to avoid. The problem is they all say different things. *Who are these people?* She asks herself. *Are they any good? Does this diet really work?* As she explores, she finds testimonials for every diet that say not only that it works, but that it works fast.

If she combines all these diets and does everything these people say is essential for MS, she'll be able to eat exactly... *nothing.* She knows for a fact she doesn't want to be one of *those people.* She cringes when she thinks about not being able to go out to eat any more. She cringes even more when she thinks about taking ten minutes to order a salad because she has to explain her very important list of what she can't have to the waiter (a list she's pretty sure will be ignored, anyway).

One thing Abby has heard a lot about in her research about good diets for people with MS is going gluten-free. *Everyone with an autoimmune disease is doing this. I'm sure it will make me feel better and lose weight,* she thinks to herself. So she cuts out gluten to see if that helps. She's been doing it really diligently for two weeks now, but she has no idea if it's working. She has no idea because when she stepped on the scale this morning, she saw that she had gained back the two pounds she lost last week.

How can other people do this so easily? What's wrong with me?

She sighs and checks her Instagram feed for a mental break. This research hurts her head. She just wants to think about something else for a while.

Within five minutes, she sees an ad on Instagram about gut flora being the key to everything. A post about how avocados can cure MS shows up as she scrolls. She sighs again. *This isn't helping.* She's already avoiding her personal messages because a friend forwarded her an article. "Thought of you!" the message said, and her friend attached a study about spinach possibly being bad for people with MS. Abby knows her friend means well but she also knows her friend didn't actually read the article before sharing it. Abby forgives her for sending something based on just the reading of a headline, but she doesn't have the energy or time right now to read another word about what she can't have.

She closes her laptop and just sits there. Frustrated, confused, annoyed. Her neurologist hasn't really helped beyond telling her that losing weight will help her MS and to eat less and move more.

She feels like a failure as she asks herself (for the thousandth time), *Why can't I figure this out?*

Feeling like she's failing is so foreign to Abby. Everyone who knows her would say she's a positive person. She believes that attitude is everything. She works very hard to see the positive in every person and situation. She starts to worry that maybe her weight is the exception to that rule.

Shaking it off, she decides that she's done with searching for the answer for now. *I have work to do. I don't have time for this now.* She welcomes the distraction of getting her files put back in her bag for work in the morning. She goes to sleep trying to be positive. Trying to believe the answer will come to her. Trying to be strong. And yet still worried that, if she can't figure out this weight thing, her future may look very different than she hopes.

Oh shit, the harsh reality hits her, *where I want to go in my life may not ever happen if I don't figure this out.*

The Missing Piece

Abby feels bounced around while she searches for an answer. As she starts to do one thing, she finds another expert saying to do something completely different. It's a rollercoaster ride she wishes would stop.

Finding your own answers can be just as frustrating. It's like standing in line at the DMV for hours, only to be told at the window that you were in the wrong line and need to start over. Then you beat yourself up for not reading the signs more carefully. It can make giving yourself breaks from focusing on weight loss seem like the kind thing to do.

There's a reason for this constant disappointment. Frustration often emerges when we're lacking in one very key element: confidence. When we're confident that we know what we're doing, we're not so insecure about being "right." You're confident you can read the words on this page. If a group of people told you that you were reading this wrong, their words wouldn't make you stop and wonder how to do it right. You probably wouldn't mind them at all. Because you're confident that you're reading this the right way.

It can be difficult to find that confidence when we keep thinking that others know better than we do. It makes sense that we feel inferior when we continue to ask other people how to make us healthy instead of asking ourselves.

How can you be assured that something is working if you don't ask the only person with firsthand knowledge about your body?

Consulted instead are the doctors, nutritionists, the internet, and the scale. You defer to experiences of other people when really you need to trust your own body.

What if we knew more about our own bodies than the experts?

How differently would you approach new information and advice? What would you think about the tiny study saying spinach is bad when you just had a spinach salad and knew you feel great? If you had that confidence – the confidence that you were the expert about your own body – you wouldn't be as likely to let bits of random information push you around into questionable territory.

But sometimes having confidence feels even more out of reach than losing weight. You may ask yourself, *How can I have confidence when nothing I do seems to be working?*

The One Thing We Know for Sure

Right now you may be as frustrated and annoyed as Abby. You may simply want to know how to lose weight. You may want someone to just *tell* you what to do.

The one thing you *can* know for sure is you are exactly where you need to be. I completely understand how ridiculous that sounds. When I was crying alone in my apartment because I'd only allowed myself to eat one grape for dessert, I would have smacked myself for saying that. But here's the thing – if I had been okay with that very restrictive diet, I would have stayed there. I would still be on it – if I didn't want more for myself (literally and figuratively). But I knew that beating myself up over one grape wasn't the answer, so I searched for more. I had the desire to find a better plan that worked for my weight loss, and for my MS. Stressing myself out over what to eat wasn't the right plan for me.

Sometimes desire looks like frustration, annoyance, even trepidation, and that's exactly where you need to be to find a better path.

Your desire has led you here, looking for a weight loss plan that works for you. You're now diving into the main source of knowledge that holds the key to being healthy: *you.*

You may not feel qualified to take that big step into the role of expert just yet, and that's okay. Small, slow steps are all you need to take your rightful place of being the authority on your health. This book is a map of steps to help you get the traction you need so your doctor visits no longer have that element of *I have to lose the weight* shame. Most importantly, you'll gain the confidence to know that your future with MS is bright and full of the adventure you crave.

Starting off, you may be a bit skeptical.

If you're like I was when I looked for the answers, you have little trust in yourself about losing weight. You may be looking back at how your weight loss has gone in the past and finding all sorts of evidence that you don't know how to do it. Or, what can feel worse, you may have proven to yourself that you *do* know what will help, but you don't have the discipline to stick with it. You may think the bottom line is what the scale says, and the scale is not being very kind to you.

These are all perfectly normal ways to feel about weight loss. We put ourselves under a lot of pressure to figure it out.

Let's Go

I was a lot like Abby. I was diagnosed with MS in 2000. I was overweight and the multiple rounds of steroids didn't help. I already had plenty of body shame around how much I weighed and, after the diagnosis, the fresh shame of having MS sat like a cherry on top. I wasn't stupid – I knew that what I ate and my lifestyle of stress and partying was abusing my body. I secretly feared that all the abuse led me to develop MS – and that everyone else was secretly thinking that, too.

When I reached the end of my rope, I looked for the answers outside of myself. Probably much like you, I wasn't happy with the answers I got. They weren't resonating with me. Whenever I followed diet advice or lifestyle recommendations, I felt like I was wearing the wrong size shoe. It looked pretty, and I wanted so badly for it to fit, but it just didn't. And that left me feeling lacking and depleted.

I did eventually find the right people who showed me the way. But they weren't diet experts, or even doctors. They were teachers, philosophers, and poets. They were the ones who told me I'd been the expert all along. They showed me how to make peace with my body and listen to it. They showed me how to tap into my own body's genius and use it to heal myself.

Just like I will show you how to heal yourself, too.

I will never have everything all figured out, and neither will you. I fully expect to have serious (organic, free range) potato chip cravings as I write this book. And that's just fine. Because the difference in me now is that I have the confidence to know that, when I do start to backslide, I can pull myself out of it way faster – and without all the heartache. I now understand how to listen to expert advice while staying true to myself – something that continues to help me discover which foods make my body sing and which don't. I'll teach you the tools that taught me what lifestyle makes my body fat melt away – so that you can find what works like that for you. I'll also show you tools I use to find that sweet spot of working out that keeps me feeling strong and vibrant – and how to adjust as I change.

The most important change is that I stopped feeling like a pinball being thrown around, thinking maybe this next person will know better than I do. I know that other people may have data that's useful, but I am the only one who has the right answer for me.

It's your time to become that person for yourself.

I understand this may feel big. It *is* big. But it doesn't have to be *scary*, and you're not doing this alone.

In these pages, I'm here as your coach, helping you through your path to finally finding the real answers. I'm not only going to show you the steps to take, but also help you with the internal struggles that may come when you take action. I'll be there with you for the doubts and the fears and will show you how to get around them and get back on course.

Not everyone with MS is seeking a solution like you are. Some are content to wait for directions on what to do. Others find more fulfillment in restating the problem than finding the solution. What you're doing takes courage. Wear that badge of honor while you go through this book, knowing that acting on your desire to get in control of your life and your MS symptoms sets you apart.

Allow me to hold your hand and answer your questions. Allow me to ask you the important questions to answer for yourself. You can do this. You were born to take control. I have no doubt.

Let's go.

⌣　⌣　⌣

Why is weight loss so confusing - especially when you have MS?

Listen to the free downloadable audio from me to get the answers to:

- What exactly is standing in my way?
- What's the real reason why traditional dieting only works for a short time?
- How can I make weight loss stick for good?

For your instant download, visit:

www.AndreaHansonCoaching.com/Learnmore.

Chapter 2

Why Is This So Important?

Where do you want to be in ten years?

What about 20?

No, this isn't a job interview, but it is an important question to answer when it comes to weight loss. Seeing your future clearly is a very important first step. If you don't know what future you want, how will you know when you get it?

Asking where you'll be in 20 years is a deliberately broad question. I will help you get more specific, but first I simply want you to think about the longevity of what you're doing. These are not quick fixes to get the weight off and then stop once you've lost enough. That's not how you get the future you want. This is about creating the *lifestyle* that works for *you*. It's about understanding that, if you do it right and do it now, this new lifestyle will impact you 10, 20, even 30+ years down the line.

Don't you love that?

Getting a clear vision of what you want is crucial. Let's shorten the time frame and take a look. In two years, where do you want to be? How do you want your body to feel? What do you want your clothes to look like? What size clothes do you want to wear? How fit do you want your body to be? How will you feel when you get up in the morning? What time do you think that would be? What will you think as you drive yourself to the neurologist's office? Or before you take your MRI? (A great way to answer these is in the present tense: "I feel" instead of "I will feel.")

Getting clear about the details of what you want for your life creates expectations of your future. Those expectations of what will happen – even if it's years from now – will influence your current actions, sometimes even unconsciously and in subtle ways. If you want to become a person who gets up at 5:00 a.m. and goes for a run, maybe you'll find yourself interested in using a beginner's running app now. Or maybe, if you want to become a person who feels confident going into an MRI, you'll start making those changes your neurologist suggests now.

When you envision the person you want to be in the future, you make different choices. But that only happens if you create a clear picture. If you're wishy-washy about how you want your life to be, you're not subtly motivated at all. Because how do you know what to do now if you don't know the result you're working toward?

Concept: Every House Has a Foundation

When you build a structure, it has a foundation. Even the tiniest of tiny houses will likely have a little concrete poured before it can be permanently placed. (I know this because a dear friend of mine is docking her Tiny House as I write this.)

The foundation anchors the structure, keeps the house insulated from outside elements, and keeps it from being flooded with moisture that would ruin what's kept inside. Foundations are important, and you need a good one for the structure of your health.

The foundation for health is creating a healthy weight. I say "creating" instead of "being" because often the path to a healthy weight creates big results in your life before you even arrive at that magic number. That's one of the beautiful things about losing weight – the benefits of health in other areas often roll in before the final goal weight is met.

What are those benefits?

Not only do losing weight and better health mean you can feel better, it can also mean numbers like cholesterol, blood sugar, blood pressure and weight all go down. This means threats of other diseases diminish and there's less worry – and less money - needing to go toward dealing with your prognosis. I don't need to explain the nitty gritty because these are benefits that we all know about. But when you have MS, these results take on a whole new meaning.

Extra weight causes inflammation. It's a normal response and it happens in everyone who's overweight. When your body has inflammation, your immune system gets excited because it wants to cure the inflammation. When there's a diagnosis like MS, the last thing you want is your immune system getting excited, because that can lead to exacerbations. So losing weight may mean lowering inflammation and, in turn, lowering the excitement level of your immune system.

Another thing that can happen while you lose weight with the steps I'll show you is that you start to pay extra attention to your body. Not just how much it weighs, but how it feels, what's normal, and when tiny changes happen that you can notice.

You will find that losing weight sets you up for that future you're now becoming clearer about. It also sets you up for a foundation of wellness and a sleeker feeling even before your natural weight is reached.

A major side effect of paying this much attention to your health and weight is that you're paying more attention to your MS. This doesn't mean you're obsessed with it. The opposite is true. You can start to control symptoms and understand them in a way that helps you address changes earlier than you would if you distracted yourself and only listened to other people.

Give me that side effect any day.

Concept: The Cycle of Success in Health

There is a growing trend in research that looks at lifestyle changes and their effects on disease and disability. I couldn't be happier that research is finally catching up. When I was first diagnosed in 2000, anyone who talked about supplements and food as a healing element for MS (or any other diagnosis) was on the fringe. Advice about this was "uncorroborated" and, therefore, very few doctors were talking about things like sunshine and minerals. I was lucky in that my neurologist was always ahead of the curve and gave me quite a few ideas from the beginning (such as taking vitamin D) that are now praised, studied, and becoming proven tools for fighting disease.

One subject on the rise in research is healthy lifestyle factors in relation to tamping down symptoms. There's even evidence showing that some diseases, like diabetes, go away entirely in some people.

This is very exciting.

No, right now there's no cure for MS. But a growing body of recent research is showing that changing certain lifestyle factors – like losing weight, exercising, eating a clean diet, and being mindful – can help quell some symptoms of MS. This is big news because what we're finding out through research is what many of us have seen firsthand all along – when you live healthfully, you have a big hand in setting yourself and your MS up for success.

This success creates a cycle of feeling confident that feeds into the motivation and consistency of making lifestyle changes. When you're able to set up this cycle, once seemingly difficult changes are made with ease, because they feed back into that cycle of confidence and success.

What This Means for You

Your bottom line probably hasn't changed. You still want to lose weight – and this highlights why the stakes are higher if you have MS. This means it's exponentially more important that attention is given to your weight *now*.

I know I'm preaching to the converted. You already want to figure out this weight thing. Now give yourself a high five for it possibly helping the prognosis of your MS as well. (I would bet you don't give yourself enough high fives for the good you're doing, so you can start with congratulating yourself for this very big deal.)

Many of my clients come to me because they know they have a history of diseases like diabetes and hypertension in their family and they don't want to develop those themselves. That's a pretty powerful motivation, and it may be a big part of what motivates you as well.

An important part of weight loss that's often brushed over is the reason *why* you're doing it. This is too big of a change to do because you want to make someone else happy, or because you're afraid of what may happen if you stay where you are. I always encourage my clients to know the positive reason of why they're making this change.

Understanding why is one place where that clear picture of your future can play a role. If that picture is clear enough, then the reason you're making these changes and paying attention to your body can be to reach that vision – especially when that vision includes delicious things like travel and grandchildren. My clear vision includes my husband and me going off the beaten path when we travel – going places where locals go. We both love that side of traveling to a new culture. Another reason for me is that I want to put our money toward retirement, instead of having to work forever to pay hospital bills. My weight loss and health are absolutely motivated by those visions.

Why you're making these changes is as important as the change itself. When you find a juicy reason why (and hopefully you'll have many), write it down on a sticky note and put it where you can read it every day. Think how it will feel when you're living that clear vision of the future, and think about why you want it. Understanding why you want to lose weight and knowing how it will feel when you get there are two big steps that give you that subtle nudge to keep going.

Let's Go

This process so far can sound intuitive. Yes, losing weight can help your MS. I'm a pretty straightforward coach, and I know that sounds simple. But if you already had the answers you need, you would be *there* – having the body and health you love, instead of *here* – wanting to find changes that work. It's great that you know there's something missing from what you're currently doing. Quite often, when someone *seems* to "figure it out," they're not doing it as well as they could, because they skip over one important piece: understanding what got you here.

Understanding what got you *here* is first.

It may feel like I'm asking you to bring up old stuff. Why you're *here* isn't really working, so why even bother looking at it? Why not go straight to the answer that will get you to *there*?

What got you *here* is not as old as you think.

The reason you're *here* is because you may believe certain things that are keeping you stuck. It's hard to see them because you often think of them as facts. But the answers to the questions I'm about to ask are simply opinions, not facts. And understanding our opinions can give us a panoramic view of why we're *here* now and not *there* already.

Answer the following questions about how you currently think. Make sure you're not answering how you thought about them "before," or using the answers you want to have.

- *What do you think about your weight loss?*
- *What do you think about your MS?*
- *What do you think about your body?*
- *How hard do you think having success and seeing results in your weight loss will be?*

Look at your answers. Are you surprised at any of them? Do you feel like they accurately portray how you think and feel about these issues? Do you feel like you're giving rote answers, or did you answer them with the ugly truth? (No one has to see these answers. I'm not asking to help anyone other than you.)

Connect with what you really believe and write the answers again if they're different. You want to see what you really believe, instead of the pretty answers you would give someone else (I have pretty answers, too) because this is a good look at why you're *here*.

Understanding what these answers really mean can help you not only get *there*, but leave *here* behind without worrying that you will come back to it as you may have in the past.

Future Focus

Let's look at that clear vision of your future. What do you want your future to look like? Most of my clients would say they want a future with independence and not having to rely on or burden their loved ones with caring for them. Taken a step farther, they say they want a future where they can travel, feel great, and not worry. You might have career ambitions or a major project you want to do someday.

Keep thinking about that future you want. If you could pluck one day out of your life 20 years from now, what would it look like?

What are you doing? How do you look and feel? Allow yourself to stop and really think about it.

Getting a clear picture of that day is priceless because it gives you an almost tangible place where you're going. Your goals are more easily reached when you have a destination in mind – not just a statistic, like "I lost 20 pounds," but an actual place and actual circumstances where you see yourself being.

If you're at the subway station, which directions will easily get you onto the right subway – "Go to the museum on Sixth Street" or "Go find the painting"? With the latter you may eventually find the right painting, but you may not know which subway line is the best, leaving you with some unexpected trips far away from the place you ultimately want to go.

When you have an actual, clear destination, you know you're on the right path. Think about that person on the subway who's confident about their destination. Who is that person and how do they act when the subway makes stops along the way? What are they thinking? Are they worried that a stop before they get to Sixth Street means they'll never arrive? Or are they confident that they will arrive at their destination no matter how many stops are along the way? How would they answer those questions I asked you in the previous section?

This is where you start shifting into the person who knows they're on the right path.

Start Where Your Are Now

One of my favorite teachers is Steven Pressfield. He has a list of accomplishments a mile long, a few of which are writing historical fiction, screenplays, and non-fiction. He's the ultimate instructor of the "get it done" mentality, and I owe much of my own professional growth to something he wrote in *Do The Work!*, his 2011 book: "Start before you're ready."

It's a beautiful statement because it summarizes why we often don't start, especially when we're a bit daunted by the work ahead of us. There are so many seemingly good reasons why we can't start in earnest to make important lifestyle changes:

- *I don't know what to do.*
- *I keep getting sabotaged – there's junk food all over the house and the office.*
- *I'm going on vacation and I can't be expected to "be good."*
- *I'll start on Monday – this weekend is already shot.*
- *I'm not ready.*

There are hundreds of "good" reasons we can come up with to not start. Have you told yourself any of these?

These excuses are part of the resistance that Pressfield talks about which slows us down. It's chatter that stops us from going after what we really want. Our opinions sound true. I'm sure a lot of these reasons sound true when you say them to yourself. After all, we wouldn't say them if they didn't seem logical.

When you start before you're ready, you skip over all of these opinions that can get in the way. If you're not worrying about being ready, excuses don't slow you down, because they no longer matter.

Think about the results you want – like looking good while you feel even better, saving money, and spending less time worrying.

Are those things you want to delay? Do you want to put them off because you're frustrated about your last snack and want to give up for a few days? Or do you want to go all in, and keep getting back on track without delay?

About five years after I was diagnosed with MS, I decided my life had way too much drama. I didn't really know what I wanted, but I continued to complain about where I was. I decided one day to stop the drama and to be less stressed. If I had waited until I was good and ready, I would never have done it. I would be in the same place now that I was ten years ago. It and I might look different, but the drama would be exactly the same. I didn't realize what I was doing, and how the drama was creating a road block to my success, until I read Pressfield's work.

Making huge changes was scary, and I didn't know if what I was doing would work. But it was exhilarating at the same time. As I made more changes and saw the positive results, I became more courageous. Just like fear begets fear, courage begets more courage.

That's exactly what happens when you "start before you're ready."

Losing weight may be a big step for you. I understand completely. Give yourself the credit you're due for jumping on that subway before you're ready to go. I promise you're packed and ready for the journey. And you're not riding alone.

Chapter 3

Not Your Mama's Diet

iet.

It's become such an ugly word. It's synonymous with *restrictions* and *hardships*. When you're on a diet, fun is not to be had. In fact, you're made to sit on the sidelines watching non-dieting people having all the fun they want, because they're allowed to eat.

Not you. You're on a diet.

It's no wonder people think they have to wait until vacation is over and any celebratory dinners are done before they can truly get into a diet. People make it hard to follow and often very restrictive because they "have" to. They're psyching themselves out before they start.

Listen to the language that's used when someone is on a diet:

- *I can't have that.*
- *I can only have a little of that.*
- *I'm not allowed to have that.*
- *Let me see if there's anything on the menu I can eat.*
- *I'm going to be bad and eat this because I really don't care.*

There's no ownership there. It's all about someone outside of you controlling what you can and can't do. It gets uncomfortable, even victimy. And stopping the diet feels like defiance, adolescent rebellion, and even resigning yourself to just not caring anymore.

No, thank you.

The truth is, diets *are* important. It's not the word *diet* that is so hated; it's the associations we give it. We hate restrictions (or see them as necessary evils), but we don't hate food. Food is an object. We can choose to eat it or not.

Let's use a definition of *diet* that's simply *what we eat*. That's it. It's what we eat. Junk food is as much a part of a diet as is being vegan. What we eat is very important. That's why we put so much stock in what nutritionists and food studies say – because we hope they have the answer to the very important question of *What food is right for me?*

Understanding the importance of finding the foods that work for your body is a cornerstone of losing weight. Exercise is great, and I'll talk more about the benefits of it in Chapter 7, but it's not the most important part of losing weight – not by a long shot. The bottom line is that if you want to lose weight, look at what you eat.

So, yes, I'm going to talk about diet because it's hugely important. But I'm not talking about restrictions or giving up control. What I'll show you is how to take *ownership* of your diet and how to start making food your choice and no one else's, ever again.

⌒   ⌒   ⌒

If you're like I was, not having anyone tell you what to do about your diet may seem foreign. When I first changed my definition of diet and started following my gut (quite literally) I felt a bit alone. I knew there wasn't going to be one diet that worked for me. I had followed too many to the T, only to find out there were aspects of them that mysteriously made me gain weight. When I realized that just because a famous guru said a certain food was the gold standard that didn't mean it was good for me, I had no crowd to follow. I was on my own.

Now I know there's so much freedom there.

When I was looking for the magic diet that worked for me, instead of feeling independent I felt confused and often betrayed. *He said avocados were so good for me, but they made me gain weight and not lose it like he said I would. Wait, I thought that food was okay to have – now he's telling me I can't have that, either?*

I was always following and never leading. I didn't think I was qualified to know how my body reacted to food. I thought I would have to get all kinds of certifications about nutrition to be able to confidently say what I could eat.

That couldn't be farther from the truth.

What I needed was to understand what worked in *my* body. Even though there are thousands of different diets, they're still either a "one size fits all" approach or filled with complicated rules. If there's one thing I've learned in 16 years of having MS, it's that there is no "one-size fits all" solution to being healthy. *Especially* when MS is involved.

We'll talk more in Chapter 6 about breaking away from the "one size fits all" mentality and finding your specific diet, but first I want to talk about food. I think food is quite possibly the most important thing you put into your body (and that includes medication).

Concept: The No-Brainer Approach to Food

Of all the different diet advice out there, common threads definitely appear. These are what I call the "no-brainers" and they're fantastic ways to make sweeping changes in your health without worrying if you're following a trend that may turn on you down the road. No-brainers focus simply on cleaning up what you currently eat.

It may be tempting to start a new diet by going gluten-, carbohydrate-, or dairy-free. I don't recommend that at first. This is probably not what you're used to hearing. But before you start looking at specific food choices for you body, it helps to be in a place where you can clearly hear your body to begin with. When we do a whole bunch of changes at once, we can miss the mark. Or, worse, we can throw the baby out with the bathwater and end up giving ourselves way more restrictions that we actually need to. For example, why go completely grain-free, when the real problem is only corn?

My hunch is that there's a lot of confusion going on in your mind and body. You may have thoughts swirling that you don't realize are affecting your drive and motivation. Hunger and emotions may be crossing paths, so that cravings and even food addictions are preventing clear communication from your body. These factors come together to create a lot of noise that stops you from truly seeing what changes work and what don't.

First, you're going to get the noise cleared out so that you can tell what's working. In order to start doing that, I suggest making some broad strokes regarding food, and I'll show you later how to fine tune.

The first broad stroke is the "no-brainer" approach to food.

We looked at changing your definition of *diet* to simply be *the food you eat*. Now let's change the definition of *food* to mean *whole ingredients in their original form*. Anything other than food in its true form is processed.

This can get tricky, because most food in stores and in our pantries is processed.

Peanut butter, olive oil, whole grain bread, and frozen broccoli – even if it's organic, grass fed, free range and made with love – is processed.

Ideally, everything we eat should be in whole, off-the-vine form. Organic and clean. Really, we should just grow everything ourselves and live off the grid. That's the only way to verify the purity of anything we eat.

Okay, let's not do that. At least not yet.

I give some processed foods a pass for now because salad dressing and salsa happen. We're human. For me, it doesn't feel good to be super nitpicky. But I still keep a close eye on where those processed ingredients originate and how they're grown.

The truth is, there's a whole layer of highly processed foods that are widely considered to be bad – even harmful – for our health. The reason they're so bad is that it's hard to say what's really in them. These are the pre-packaged foods that have ingredient lists two inches long, containing words you can't pronounce and that you may also have seen listed in your stain remover. These are bars, cereals, frozen dinners, and food from not-so-high-end restaurants. There are some scary ingredients in what are called "ultra-processed" foods, and they often have a higher amount of sugar, and sodium that you can't even taste.

There are too many studies to count that link sugar and too much sodium to health issues and inflammation in the body. By simply cutting out these ultra-processed foods, your sugar and sodium consumption (not to mention your chemical intake) will go way down.

I spent many years feeling pissed off and out of control whenever I restricted my diet to lose weight, but I now see that the real place I had no control was when I ate ultra-processed foods. I thought I was exercising total control because I was "eating what I want," but the irony is that I wasn't controlling the amount of crap that was entering my body during those times of "freedom."

Another great way to start cleaning up your food is by not eating sugar. If you're already doing well with staying away from processed foods, releasing sugar is a great place to go next. This is a big change I've made in my life and, to be honest, I wouldn't have believed all the benefits if they weren't happening to me. Weight loss, definitely, but my triglyceride levels (a type of fat stored in blood, too much of which can elevate the chances of stroke and heart disease) are miniscule, my energy levels are super high, and my mind is clear. These are effects I felt within a week of quitting sugar. To be clear, this includes sugar and also any sugar substitutes, such as high-fructose corn syrup, artificial sweeteners, sugar substitutes – even the natural kind. I eat whole fruit, but rarely drink fruit juice (only if it's cold-pressed and juiced within hours of drinking it). Again, we're talking about food very close to its original form.

Quitting sugar is a big change to make – I still can't believe I drink coffee and tea with no sweetener – but it's given me one of the highest payoffs of anything I've done.

◡ ◡ ◡

These are great places to start cleaning up your diet. I suggest doing one of them at a time, even though they will eventually piggy-back on each other, and the second change will be easier after the first. Pacing yourself is important, because these are big steps. Later in this chapter, I'll give you a tool to help you with pacing.

Case Study: Mary

I had been working with Mary for a few weeks before she opened up about her habit. Everyday after dropping her son off at soccer practice, she swung by the drive-thru and got a shake. She described the shake to me in detail, and I could hear her craving it while we were on the phone. "This isn't just any shake," she said. "It's cookies and cream, with the best vanilla custard, and just the right amount of chocolate. They use real chocolate syrup, too. You can tell the difference, you know."

She then became aware of how caught up she was in the description of her shake, and went on to say how much shame she felt around that habit, and that she didn't feel in control of it at all.

"I swear, my car just auto-pilots over there," she said and nervously laughed.

Her nervous laughter didn't come because I got mad or lectured her. She wasn't afraid of what I would say. She was feeling her own disapproval.

Mary may have made fun of herself driving home with her shake – she may have even defended it while laughing nervously. The truth was she hated that loss of control. She wished she didn't "have to" visit the drive-thru, and she felt like it was an addiction. She even quoted a passage she'd read online about how sugar is an addiction that's like heroin. I agreed with her, up to a point – I still do.

Sugar is addictive. But the addiction is not insurmountable.

What Mary and I worked together on in the next few weeks of coaching sessions was helping her quit the addiction. We started with why she had it in the first place and what she thought of it. We explored everything she thought was facts and why those thoughts were holding her in place. She learned how to release those belief systems and tag them for easy detection when they came up again. We talked and walked her through the ups and downs of leaving a sugar habit behind.

Mary kicked and screamed and cried. It was hard for her, especially when she re-ignited her taste for sugar by having "just one." But she did enough self-exploration to be able to take ownership of her actions and act in a way that was healthier and that she wanted more than she wanted the sugar. She was so proud of herself and pleased with the results.

That kick-started her weight loss and her feelings of freedom with food. At the beginning of our time together she would swear that it was eating what she wanted that meant freedom in her diet. By the end of our sessions, Mary she said that having control was the ultimate freedom.

What This Means for You

There is so much blame to go around when it comes to food. We can blame the manufacturers for using addictive chemicals. We can blame the marketers for using skinny people to make junk food look so healthy and light. We can blame our own chemistry for allowing behaviors like addiction to happen. We can blame the food scientists for crafting the right combination of chemicals to entice our natural biology to crave it. We blame time for not being long enough to let us plan ahead better, or our schedules for not permitting us to really pay attention. We blame other people for putting "bad" food in front of us when we're hungry. Often, we blame ourselves for being "weak," for having no willpower, and for "not getting into gear."

The truth is, who's to blame for the food you eat is old news, because *it doesn't matter*. What you ate even earlier today is done. Assigning blame is a waste of time and energy. Even if you're blaming yourself, feeling like you're failing doesn't serve you.

What's a better use of the time and energy you get back when you stop focusing on blame? Making simple, no-brainer choices about your food – starting with your very next meal.

You have way more control than you likely give yourself credit for. Even if you do feel addicted to sugar or chemicals in your food, you have the final say.

You *can* do this.

Let's Go

Pacing yourself is an essential part of getting started. I want to give you a tool that can help you both see where you are right now and help you decide on the first changes you'll make that will help with pacing.

But first, a public service announcement: food journals are not bad. Just like diets, and food, they have received a bad rap because we assign them all of these negative associations. If you beat yourself up about what food you eat, you will hate food journaling. If you feel scared of what you'll discover when you journal, because you think eating certain foods makes you inherently "good" or "bad," you will hate food journaling. If you want to focus only on moving forward and completely changing your diet, without looking at what you currently eat, you will hate food journaling.

I invite you to have a different definition of the food journal. This is not about beating yourself up. It's not about dreading what you've already eaten. A food journal is just *information*.

If you're scared to do this, hate that I'm even suggesting it, or are already planning on skipping this step and moving to the next chapter, I ask that you please do something first: ask yourself why you don't like the idea of keeping a food journal. Your list of reasons is pure gold because it gives you a good idea of the stigma you're placing on it, and it also provides proof that it's not the food journal that makes you feel this way. Plus, you haven't started using my version of a food journal yet. The reason you feel this way is because you're thinking about food journaling in a certain way, not because of the actual journal. And thoughts can be changed.

Keeping that in mind, I ask that you give the food journal a try for one week. The reason I say one week is because that's typically how long it takes to get over the Observer Effect and have a good baseline.

The Observer Effect happens when the object (in this case the behavior of eating) being studied changes simply because it's being watched. I have no doubt this is a very real phenomenon when it comes to food journals.

Start by tracking the time of day you eat and what you eat. You can do this in any format you like – some of my clients take pictures of what they eat so they remember everything.

That's all you need to do for the first week of your food journal. No changes to your diet – just observe the status quo. If you feel any resistance to this, or find yourself omitting certain things (it's ok – we all do it), notice what you're thinking and write it down. I'll show in a later chapter how we'll use that to help you.

Future Focus

When you start your food journaling as pure observation (and not beating yourself up), a major shift in awareness happens. You see what's currently happening and you begin to map out how you want to change your lifestyle to get the future that you want. This is where you can bring awareness to playing around with what "no-brainers" you can change first in your food. It's also where you can see how far you want to go at first (do you cut out all processed food, for example, or just the ones with certain chemicals at first?).

You have all the control over where you start and how much you do – and, with your food journal, you have a great visual on how to pace yourself. As you begin to make changes, you'll be able to tell, for example, if you're changing 10% of your food choices or 100%. How much change gives you the highest possibility of staying with it? How much change will make you quit on week two?

Use this beginning status quo food journal to prepare to map it out.

Getting really good at this step of food journaling for observation will help you not only at the beginning, but anytime you would like to recalibrate to get more specific with your diet. You're getting into the role of looking at your life as a scientist would: documenting status quo and seeing how changes fit.

I use this status quo food journaling whenever I want to up-level my health, like when I want to try different foods or pinpoint something I don't think is working. This is a skill that will always be useful as you up-level your health as well.

In order for food journaling to be a useful tool for you, pay special attention to the stigma you're currently giving it. Getting over that piece first is essential.

Start Where You Are Now

Whenever I start looking at a client's food and what they're currently doing, it's always important to lead with kindness. In no way is this looking for an excuse to beat yourself up or blame yourself for where you are now. Anger has no place when you're moving forward, and assigning blame only holds you back.

It's time to get ahead. It's time to make the changes you know can directly help your health and also help your MS. But it's important that you have your own back this whole time by being kind to yourself. That's the only way to make changes that stick.

I've white-knuckled changes in my diet and exercise, forcing myself to do what someone else outlined for me while blaming myself handily for getting fat. I assure you that doesn't work. My hunch is that you know this firsthand, too.

Give yourself a chance and do these steps with kindness this time. Notice when you're fighting with yourself and when you feel guilt or shame. If you start to look at your *diet* as simply *the food you eat*, you will see options for change that you may not have otherwise seen.

You might even leave room to be pleasantly surprised.

⌣　⌣　⌣

What's the easiest way to find out what food does (and doesn't) work for you?

Get the free instant downloadable audio from me and find out. Visit **www.AndreaHansonCoaching.com/Learnmore.**

Chapter 4

Hungry for More

Think back to the last time you ate.

It doesn't matter if you ate an entire meal or a handful of something tasty. Imagine yourself back in that moment right before you ate it.

What did you eat? Chapter 3 rules still apply – this is not about shaming yourself if you had an entire bar of white chocolate. It's not even about congratulating yourself if you had half a serving of 95% dark chocolate. Whatever you ate, it was only food. Think about what that food was.

Why did you eat it? If the first answer that comes to mind is "I don't know," give yourself a moment to really think about the reason you ate. There is always a reason why we do anything, and knowing the motivation for your actions gives you a huge advantage. Your motivation could have been that you were hungry or bored or even nervous about something. Maybe something tasty was on the counter looking lonely and you couldn't resist. It could be that you were starving because you skipped breakfast this morning.

There are any number of reasons why we eat.

When I started getting curious about why I ate, I was shocked to find out all of my motives. I would eat when I was stressed out, because being full made me feel calmer. I would eat when I was unsure about something, because eating was one thing I could always be sure about. I would eat when I wanted to think about something else, because nothing distracted me like a big plate of home-style food (and then the ensuing drama about what I just ate and how out of control I was that came after that last bite). Being hungry was only one of my motives for eating.

In later chapters, I'll discuss other reasons why we eat when we're not hungry and how to stop those reasons from clouding judgments about what to eat. You may have your own list of why you eat that has nothing to do with actually needing nutrients from food.

But focusing first on genuine hunger is essential. Because it's not until you can separate genuine hunger from all the other reasons you eat that you'll be able to easily identify those other factors that are getting in the way of eating the way you would like to.

Concept: Genuine Hunger

How do you know when you're hungry?

Think about all the signs you get that help you know it's time to eat. This is a tricky question that often isn't explored. You may take it for granted that your stomach grumbling or your brain getting foggy are the obvious ways you know that you need food.

What else happens?

My clients often say they just *know* it's time to eat. For example, many say they get hunger pains, and feel light-headed. Others get insistent when it's time to eat: "I *have to have food* or my blood sugar drops and I get woozy."

When I was really hungry I would have a wave of confusion come over me and aggressively want something to eat. Thinking about fasting for a blood test would make me really nervous about what might happen.

I've heard it all: headaches, cramps, confusion, fatigue, the body simply shutting down, and a strong drive to eat immediately – no room for negotiation. Having this type of hunger can lead to eating what's right in front of you if you don't feel like there's time to make a better choice. Hunger can bring out the worst in people. When we're hungry, making a good decision about what to eat often goes out the window.

What if I told you that having pains or insecurity about being hungry aren't really signs of hunger?

I completely understand the opposition to this. I've had clients who were usually sweet as pie completely lose it when I suggest there's nothing wrong with being hungry. They would swear up and down that they'd have to call for an ambulance if they couldn't eat every few hours. (And none of them had a disease that mandated eating food that often.)

We can get very insecure about hunger. Before they learn about genuine hunger, my clients tend to eat before they're hungry if there's a projected amount of time they'll be without food. The thought of being hungry in the future would drive them to fill up their stomachs ahead of time.

This is fear-based hunger that is, in part, driven by the effects of eating the wrong foods (largely processed food and sugar). Our bodies are telling us something, but they're not telling us that we're actually hungry.

Dr. Joel Fuhrman, who wrote the book *Eat To Live*, first cued me in to how our bodies actually communicate hunger. He taught me that what he calls "true hunger" is felt in the throat, and delivers no feelings of insecurity. When I learned this, my whole viewpoint of hunger changed.

Naturally, I played around with how hunger felt in my body. (I eagerly use myself as a guinea pig for all the tools and concepts I teach.) I detailed in my food journal what I thought was hunger, and then, as I cut out processed foods and other foods that my body didn't like, I noticed how dramatically what I had thought was hunger changed. After only a few days, gone was the insecurity about being hungry. A few weeks after stopping ultra-processed foods, I realized that I was able to function quite well while I was hungry. I was astonished to find that I could carry on normally and that the world did not, in fact, end because I was late eating lunch. I even became *that person* I would have sworn I could never be – I sometimes forgot to eat.

Genuine hunger is felt in the throat. It's felt in the mouth, with more saliva being created. There's nothing insecure about it. We can function for long periods of time while being hungry. Genuine hunger doesn't change our mood. Genuine hunger is simply communication from our body telling us it's ready for food when we are.

Understanding real hunger was life-changing for me and provided a feeling of control that helped me to not only stay the course and lose weight but also to become more in tune with my body's constant communication.

Case Study: Jenny

It was my second session with Jenny and she was considering the same question that I asked you earlier: "How do you know when you're hungry?"

"Um… I don't know," she said after a moment.

"Think about it for a bit," I encouraged. "How did you know it was time for lunch today?"

"It was noon." She said flatly. "It was time to eat."

I probed a bit farther. "How did your body feel?"

"My stomach was growling a little, I guess." She answered. "I don't know. The normal stuff."

Jenny using the clock to tell her when she needed to eat is a great illustration of a common issue. Looking at something completely outside of yourself, like what time it is, to judge if your body is ready for food means you're missing the signs your body gives you. If you're focused on the wrong signs, you're missing the right ones.

As I continued working with Jenny, she learned how to pay attention to her body and the different ways it communicated genuine hunger to her. She had blocked the signs because she didn't realize how relevant they were. All she knew was if she stuck to an eating schedule, she felt better. But the reason she felt better on that schedule wasn't because she gave her body what it needed, it was because that schedule kept her feeling full. Her eating schedule never left room for being hungry, because she thought being hungry was bad. She had never allowed herself the freedom of knowing that hunger isn't something to fear. As we worked together, she began to use actual hunger as an important tool for helping her to know if she was eating the best way possible for her body.

I'll break this to you as gently as I can – the clock has no idea when your body needs nutrients and fuel. The clock doesn't know you. It hasn't met your family or posted on your Facebook feed. If even you aren't 100 percent sure when your body is hungry, how can a household object know?

Your body holds the wisdom of when you're genuinely hungry. If you pay attention, you'll find that your body uses very clear signs. What makes these cues difficult to understand are factors like being disconnected with your body, and eating foods that your body doesn't love, because that creates events in your body that you confuse with hunger, such as light-headedness and weakness.

What This Means for You

Understanding your hunger is essential. Hunger in its truest form can give us so much information. We all have different metabolisms and different ways we process food. Some people do really well with wild game meat, but for others the right protein is fish. Some people need to eat every three hours, while others do better fasting at different times during the day. There are questions around not only specific foods, like different grains, but also amounts of foods, like how much fat to include in your diet. Figuring out what makes you fire on all cylinders goes beyond food to what exercise is best for you right now, and knowing the signs that help you and your doctor figure out what supplements you need. There are seemingly endless questions to ask yourself, and if you're not cued in to your body's communication, you stay confused about how to find what's right for you.

Pain, digestive sounds and movements, dizziness, restlessness, saliva output, and weakness are all ways our body talks to us. When we misinterpret those signs as "just hunger" and muffle them by filling our stomachs with food, we miss the chance to understand what's happening on a deeper and more useful level. Instead of hunger, those could be signs that our body's having a hard time digesting something. What we think is our stomach growling for food could be our body trying to get rid of the effects of something we ate earlier that was bad for us. What if we ate something that caused inflammation and the body's response to suppress the danger takes the form of cravings which we misinterpret as hunger. Then we're in danger of eating more of what we should be staying away from.

Hunger is way more than just knowing how much and when to eat.

This whole process of taking control of your wellbeing is all about you becoming proficient in what works best for *you* to be as healthy as possible. In order to do that, you need to be able to separate hunger from all the other noise that keeps you from truly hearing from your body about what diet and, ultimately, what lifestyle works for you.

How do you know you're feeling hungry? How often do you feel hunger? Hopefully you've already started thinking about your answers.

The very best place to start is by understanding how hunger works in *your* body.

Let's Go

This chapter has outlined many ways people think they feel hunger, but it's time to start looking at your own ways your body tells you you're hungry. There may be ways that I haven't touched on that you're thinking hunger shows up for you.

Here's a simple exercise to help you find out the details of your own hunger: Set aside five to ten minutes before every time you eat. Before you take a bite, sit quietly for a moment. Closing your eyes may help you to focus. Think about your answers to the following questions:

- *How does my stomach physically feel right now?* Describe the sensation in detail. Is it hot or cold? Do you feel movement or is it still? Does it feel angry or calm?
- *How does my throat feel right now?* Again, describe it in detail.
- *How does the rest of my body feel?* Scan your body from head to toe to see how each part feels.
- *How does my whole body feel right before I eat?* Summarize the physical feelings.

When you do this every time you eat, you'll start to get an accurate picture of what you're labeling as hunger. In the next chapter, we'll go over how emotions play a role in hunger. For now, only focus on the physical sensations in your body.

If you're having a hard time focusing for five to ten minutes before you eat, that's ok. Try to focus for as long as you can. Any amount of information you can get here is golden.

The best way to do this is to write down what you find. You only need to write a few lines before each meal. This will help you see patterns in how you feel before you eat.

Get a good understanding of how your hunger feels to you now. Then, as you change your diet, you can better see how your feeling of hunger changes. You'll see how different your hunger feels once you start to eliminate foods like sugar.

Future Focus

When you're practiced at knowing your feeling of genuine hunger, a whole world opens up to you. As you go though life with this awareness, you'll constantly notice how your body feels. This awareness will become second nature to you and being tapped in to how your body feels won't be nearly as labored as it feels right now.

Once you get through these first steps of eliminating the "no-brainer" foods (discussed in Chapter 3), you'll move on to looking at other foods that you may want to incorporate or take out of your diet. This is the fine-tuning portion that will be a part of and affect your life-long health. As you age and change, your body will, too. When you understand genuine hunger, you have an easy way to notice changes in your body, including changes in what your body needs. If you're used to feeling genuine hunger, but all of a sudden notice you're getting that urgency again around eating, that's your cue to look more closely at what you're eating and to question if it's still good for you.

This is a life-long skill that will serve you well.

When you become comfortable with hunger, you'll have a healthy relationship with food. No longer labeling food as "good" or "bad," and taking the drama out of eating, can make cutting out certain foods not such a big deal.

Have you ever eaten out with someone who's obviously lamenting being gluten-free? They pine after bread and talk about how they don't get that "full" feeling without it. They become "that person" who complains about the food restrictions. Finding what your genuine hunger feels like and taking steps to eliminate the foods that your body doesn't like will help you keep from being "that person." When you know firsthand that your body doesn't like a food, not eating it won't be a big deal. In fact, it will feel more like kindness than restriction.

Sounds pretty freeing, doesn't it?

Start Where You Are Now

Changing your diet to find that special combination of foods that works for you can be complex. That's why meticulously going through these first steps is essential. Once you stop eating the "no-brainer" foods and begin food journaling to practice your observation skills, and understand your genuine hunger, the dominos of finding foods that work and don't work can fall into place.

But beginnings can be tough.

When I first started noticing my genuine hunger, it felt like little ants running all over my stomach. As I sat with that sensation, it got bigger and bigger. I was so uncomfortable that I had to eat – and quickly – so the sensation would go away. At first I could sit and feel my hunger for maybe 30 seconds. I was so proud of myself for paying attention for that long. I would excuse myself from the table and go sit in the bathroom for just a moment of quiet, and pay attention to my body. I won't lie – it was intense in the beginning. But I did it. And sitting with that sensation unlocked not only what my genuine hunger felt like but also led to finding out more than what food could tell me.

I'll share what that sensation of ants in my stomach really was later on (hint: it had nothing to do with food). But know that I understand how hard these first steps can be. You've been eating to avoid these sensations for a reason. Pulling back the comfort of feeling full and taking a look for the first time at being hungry can be scary.

I assure you there's nothing to be afraid of.

This is the front line of why you're eating food that you know isn't good for you, or why you're eating too much and too often. This is also where you can stop feeling like these sensations are holding you hostage.

You can do this. Once you get used to sitting with your hunger for five to ten minutes, the rest won't seem so bad.

◡ ◡ ◡

Our genuine hunger can be tangled with so many factors.

With your free audio comes a complimentary phone call with me.

You can ask me any questions you like and we'll talk about precisely how to learn your body's hunger signals over time.

Snag your free audio and complimentary call with me by visiting:

www.AndreaHansonCoaching.com/Learnmore.

Chapter 5

Why We Do Anything

S everal diet gurus have given me "the exact plan that will work," and I've followed them all faithfully. A few of those plans were from gurus I met with personally; other plans were from a book or an online program. I've definitely put in my time when it comes to diets and health plans. With some plans, I did lose a lot of weight. But however much weight I lost came right back, and then some. That's because even the most detailed of "do exactly as I say" plans were missing the crucial components that turn a flash in the pan diet into a consistent lifestyle.

As I was forcing myself to make ambitious changes (and failing), the fact that the plans were missing something wasn't even a thought in my mind. I always thought the problem was me.

You don't know what you don't know.

I thought I wasn't disciplined enough. I would cry about why I lacked the willpower to keep going. I ached to know why I sabotaged myself instead of sticking to the plan that I could clearly see was helping me lose weight.

I thought I was working against myself for some sad reason that I couldn't figure out.

Talking to my then diet mentors didn't help. I was told to "keep going," and that of course it's hard, but I have to be tough. My favorite comment I got from a trainer was, "Pain is weakness leaving your body." He was a retired Marine.

We often find the answers to one problem when we're looking at something entirely different.

I had known that my stress levels were over the top. Between my MS, fear of a future with MS symptoms, my job in finance (and all the office drama that comes with it), and my almost lifelong weight struggle (which existed in my head even when my body wasn't overweight), you can imagine that my stress was out of control. I thought my biggest problem was my stressful job. While looking for a new one, I discovered the world of coaching. Coaching showed me that the problem had nothing to do with my job. Diving into coaching not only taught me the real reasons why I was stressed out, but also the reasons why the diet plans I had tried weren't sticking.

Those plans weren't addressing what I was *thinking* or the emotions that came up for me as I made and tried to make big changes.

What we think and how we feel drive our actions. It's no wonder I was having a hard time staying focused. My thoughts and emotions were not in line with the actions I wanted to take.

Many programs try to "coach" by holding people accountable so they stick with the work. But thinking you need someone else to make you work is disempowering. It may be effective for short bursts, but it's hard (and expensive) for someone else to "make" you work at something for the rest of your life.

Many plans try to address thoughts and feelings by telling participants how important it is to stay positive, no matter what. What that does is create a positivity that is white-knuckled along with the diet changes, only to crash in a fit of "I don't care" setbacks.

A lifetime of health is almost never created with tough love approaches.

Having a deep understanding of what you're feeling and what you're thinking is essential if you want to make true changes that last. You've already started to gain awareness of what you're truly thinking by answering the questions I asked in the first four chapters. And we'll take an even deeper dive into your thoughts in Chapter 10.

For now, let's look at emotions and how they relate to our weight and our health, and how they can make or break our desired changes.

Whether you've already identified your emotional connection with food or not, it exists. But there's nothing to fear. These are simply emotions. They may feel like the big monster behind the curtain, but I assure you they're just smoke and mirrors once you pull that curtain back.

Concept: Why We Do Anything

Emotions can get a bad name. Sometimes they're trite, sometimes they're too big to handle. They can get in the way, or show up when we least expect them. We can get teased for having them, and sometimes wish we didn't have them at all. The "good" emotions can seem fleeting while the "bad" ones seem to stick around too long. We hear about the power of positive emotions and are told the negative ones don't help us.

Do you want the real scoop on emotions?

First, they're not positive or negative. They're simply reactions to thoughts, and they're accompanied by physical changes in our bodies, like a lump in our throat when we're sad, or laughter that seems to burst out of us. When emotions are felt all the way through, they subside very quickly.

Sadness doesn't have a hold on us anymore than happiness does. The difference is that most times we allow our happiness to be expressed at 100 percent, yet we only allow our sadness to be expressed at maybe 50 percent. That's why happiness seems to go away and sadness sticks around. We still have a large percentage of sadness suppressed inside, waiting to get out.

If we allowed the "ugly cry" as much as we allowed the "hysterical laughter," we wouldn't feel so afraid of the sadness never going away.

Emotions are not the enemy. Some clients who feel like emotions have a death grip on them challenge me on this point.

That's often because emotions are being confused with diagnosed disorders like clinical depression or anxiety. A diagnosed disorder implies that there is chemical or physical change in the brain, so these feelings are no longer pure emotions. They're disorders and have a very different effect on us than simply feeling sad. Emotions can be felt and let go of, but changes in the brain that cause disorders need further treatment.

The second thing about emotions is that they're why we do everything. Every single action is taken because we think it will make us feel better.

I *know*. It sounds way too simple, doesn't it?

Test it.

Why are people nice to strangers? Because it feels good.

Why do you want to make your loved ones happy? Because it makes you happy when they're happy.

Why do people hate to be late? Because they're uncomfortable when they show up and everyone looks at them.

Why are people less than excited to keep a food journal? Because they feel embarrassed or even ashamed to look at what they've been eating.

When you're taking any action, stop and ask yourself why you're doing it. If you dig deep enough for that answer it will show that you're taking action to either feel something good, or to avoid feeling something bad.

Avoiding emotions is a big reason why we eat when we're not hungry, or eat foods we know aren't healthy. *We're avoiding a feeling.* Often we're avoiding "negative" feelings, but sometimes we're trying to avoid "positive" ones as well.

The bottom line is that your emotions need to be felt in order to gain comfortable control of your weight.

Case Study: Amy

Amy was really frustrated as she described her weight. "I don't understand it. I'm doing everything I can. I eat healthy all day but the scale isn't moving."

We looked at her previous day's food to see what was going on. She recounted a near perfect list of food and portion sizes. An A+ in eating.

"Then, of course, when I get home from work I have to eat a snack." She adds, "But usually it's popcorn with no butter."

"How are you eating this popcorn?" I ask, sensing something worth exploring.

"It's a pre-popped bag from the store that's organic. I just grab the bag and have my snack while I'm watching the news. I need to put my feet up and rest after working all day."

"How often do you do this?"

"Like… every day," she said, her voice sounding less upbeat than a few minutes ago. "I try to have something healthier instead, but I'm seriously hungry. Once I start eating, the bag is gone before I know it."

By then she had put together just how *much* of a snack she was having.

It was a lot. And she felt out of control with the popcorn.

She wasn't lying – all day she ate really well – but at the end of the day when she got home she was more than hungry. She was starving. The kind of starving that has you eating five servings of popcorn and still craving more.

What I recognized as I talked with Amy was that it most likely wasn't only hunger she was feeling. You may remember from the previous chapter that hunger is doable. It doesn't stop you from functioning. You can go about your day feeling hungry.

If you don't feel like you can function without eating, something else is going on.

For Amy, that something else was emotional.

All day at work, she was distracted. She managed a large group and there were always issues and people in her office, emails and meetings. Lunch was often eaten on the go. She had no time to digest anything – especially emotions.

When she got home, there were a few hours before she had to start dinner and everyone else came home, bringing more distractions. In that time when she was alone, all of those feelings she had been distracted from during the day came bubbling up. But she didn't want to feel them. So she ate instead. Watching the news and munching on popcorn was yet another distraction. Which is also why she felt like she couldn't stop doing it. The second she did, those emotions that she would rather not deal with would come up.

That explained why she felt unhinged by the end of the day, when all her distractions were gone. It also explained why she was still starving after she had more than a few servings of popcorn. It wasn't hunger she was feeding. It was her effort to distract herself from how she was really feeling.

We began to untangle what she was feeling and why she was distracting herself. She started to identify her emotions and understand how to deal with them in more healthy and supportive ways. Once she was able to see how her hunger could be emotional, we started putting what she needed in place to feed the emotional hunger instead.

Amy's work was in learning how to feel validated and like she was enough. She was a strong person with huge ambitions, but the MS had left a part of her feeling like she didn't measure up and that rejection would catch up to her eventually. Popcorn would never make that feeling go away, but understanding her emotions and facing them head on did.

What This Means for You

For some people, following a diet plan is effortless. They never feel like they're missing out because they can't eat cheese. If you're reading this book, following a diet may not be that easy for you. That's completely okay. It wasn't that simple for me, either.

The good news is uncovering *why* you struggle with food can give you an advantage that extends beyond your diet.

Our emotions are systemic. You may see them manifested in your weight, but they can also show up without us realizing in our relationships, our jobs, how we treat ourselves, in other areas of health, and in how we are with our kids. By connecting with why you struggle with food, you're figuring out something that goes way beyond your weight.

When Amy discovered that the real reason she was tearing through popcorn was that she felt like she didn't measure up, a light bulb came on. She saw how she was a little graspy with her husband's affection and how she felt needy for attention from her teenage daughter. She even felt jealous of people at work who she thought weren't even on the same playing field as her. Strange behaviors started to make sense for Amy when she realized her emotions were running unmanaged in the background of her mind.

Now is a great time to look into what emotions show up and how they're affecting you. The effect may blatantly show up in your eating, but those emotions are at work in other areas of your life, too.

Let's Go

The last chapter was about starting to notice how hunger feels for you – how it feels in your stomach and throat, for example.

Let's add a layer to that.

Now that you've asked yourself a few times how you feel physically regarding being hungry, you can start to distinguish between genuine hunger and emotional hunger. Remember, genuine hunger is felt in your throat. Your salivation increasing and your body having a sense that it's time to eat are signs that your hunger is genuine. But when you feel hunger pains, an urgency to eat, and restlessness when you take a moment to feel, that's most likely emotional hunger.

If you're following this program and doing the exercises in the chapters, you've already been cutting out major toxins in your diet, such as sugar or ultra-processed food. So hunger resulting from foods your body is rejecting should be subsiding.

As you're sitting for that brief period before you eat, notice how your body feels. Notice everything from the top of your head to your feet and describe the physical sensations.

Now start asking yourself these additional questions:

- *What part of how I'm feeling is likely genuine hunger?*
- *What emotion am I feeling right now?*
- *How does that emotion feel physically in my body?*

Adding these questions to your brief routine before you eat will help you distinguish hunger from emotions. Your answers will also help you start to identify what emotions you're actually feeling.

If you're still having trouble sitting for a full ten minutes while you uncover how you're feeling, I encourage you to do what you can to keep it up. Add more time little by little. The longer you can sit and identify what you're feeling emotionally and how you feel it in your body, the better. What you're starting to do is allow yourself to *feel* these emotions. By allowing them, they can subside. You will start to find that, in the instances where you know it isn't genuine hunger, inquiring about your emotions will take the urgency out of how you feel and you may not even be hungry anymore.

Be patient with yourself as you add this piece to the puzzle. Stick with it as long as you can and you'll find out some amazing things about yourself that you never knew.

Future Focus

When you start to tease out the feelings of genuine hunger from emotional hunger, you start to solve the puzzle of how our body works and what it needs to be healthy. As you practice this and become better at it, you won't need ten minutes by yourself in order to focus any more. You'll be able to do it in an instant. You'll be able to tell in the moment why you're craving that donut. You'll know if that craving comes from feeling upset about a conversation you had earlier, if you had sugar the other day and your body is still feeling slightly addicted, or if you're genuinely hungry – in which case, you'll have the choice to choose something other than a donut and that will likely feel pretty easy.

Having this barometer at your fingertips is priceless.

Imagine being able to process your feelings of guilt or anxiety while sitting in a meeting. No one knows that you're letting those emotions run through your body. No one is aware of how you're feeling, because you're just sitting there, relaxing while you allow it. Imagine being able to resolve drama with someone way faster.

Imagine no longer mindlessly eating a box of crackers because you feel nervous about an MRI.

Being proficient at this skill has a ripple effect that will change your future. Yes, this skill is that powerful. Those times when you felt out-of-control hunger and didn't know why you ate food that you knew was bad for you were due in large part to how you felt emotionally. Getting ahead of your emotions and making them a non-issue when it comes to eating can change food forever.

This is how you strengthen your relationship with yourself and stop overeating.

Start Where You Are Now

Beautiful things happen when you learn to sit with your emotions. You may be like me and have to sit with your fear first. When I had that feeling like ants were crawling around in my stomach it was straight up fear. I was afraid I was going to "lose it." I assumed that "losing it" meant I would go crazy – unless I ate that seven-layer dip. Then I'd be okay.

My fear that I was going to "lose it" was manifesting in my stomach, feeling like ants crawling faster and faster and covering a larger area in my body the longer I left it. It sounds dramatic, and it was. At first, being afraid of that feeling of fear kept me from being able to sit very long and feel it.

When I did pay attention before I ate, I started by identifying that the sensation was not, in fact, genuine hunger. I admitted that food would only make the sensation go away temporarily and it would be back sooner or later. Eventually I was able to label what I was feeling and see that it was fear that made my body feel that way, but feeling that emotion, calmly, made it subside rather quickly. Now I know that my fear of "losing it" was exactly that. Fear of what would happen when I lost the weight.

That's what you may find as well. The act of suppressing emotions keeps us from finding the real reasons we don't want to do something. I didn't want to lose weight because I was afraid of who I would become once I wasn't "the fat friend" anymore. I was afraid that my MS still wouldn't be better and all of my efforts would be for naught. I was afraid of stepping out of the cocoon of my body weight, because it kept me from my full potential, and though that cocoon was unsatisfying, it was safe, nonetheless.

If you're finding fears, be patient with yourself. Keep showing kindness as you sit for as long as you can to figure out what type of hunger you're feeling and what emotions you're feeling. This is a very vulnerable spot to be in. It's likely you've been covering up your feelings and your vulnerability pretty well so far.

But if you want a strong relationship with yourself, the kind where you know what to eat and how to be healthy, the kind where you're in charge and confident while you find that unique plan that works for you – then feeling emotions is an essential step.

Understanding your emotions may take longer than you would like, if you're doing this on your own. Whether you do work on your own or with a coach, know that it's worth every minute you put into it.

Chapter 6

The Body Connection

W hat if your body could write you a full report detailing exactly what it needs in order to be healthy? That would be the essay to end all essays. It would include everything you asked for in one neatly bound file (because you know your body would dig office supplies). It would include whether you should go vegan or stick with meat, whether you should stay away from gluten or dairy – or eat both, what makes your skin break out, and the run-down on what supplements you need. You would also learn why you're so stressed out about some things and completely chill about others.

Would you want a copy of that report?

Of course you would. You would immediately stop reading this book and start studying that one, highlighter in hand.

But would you use that information?

Think about that one for a second. Would you trust what the report said? Or would you think it was too good to be true? Would you use the information if it differed from what the "experts" said?

What if your body's report told you that wheat, dairy, and gluten were good for you? Would that make you pause, since that goes against current advice and trends?

Here's the truth: *you already have this report*. Unfortunately your body can't use office supplies to neatly bind it for you, so it may not look how you imagined. But your body does give you access to what the report says – on a daily and a moment-to-moment basis.

The hard part is that the information isn't written in words. Your body's messages come in pictures, physical feelings, and emotions.

Now that you're becoming aware of how you're physically feeling, and of the differences between your genuine hunger and emotional hunger, it's time to pull those pieces together and learn how to listen to the information *your* body has.

All the diet plans out there are based on other people's bodies.

My hunch is that, until now, you've been giving those diets, proven by other people's bodies, credence over what you own body knows. That's perfectly understandable. Their marketing is great, and the common logic is that the experts know more about food and the human body than you do. And that may be true on some level, but what you may be figuring out as you go through this book is that although experts may have knowledge you're looking for, they aren't the final word.

You are.

Concept: What Your Body Has Been Telling You All Along

Have you ever had a gut feeling about someone you just met? You don't know *how* you know it, but you're sure that you two are kindred spirits. You click, and hanging out with them is fun and effortless.

How do you know what your gut feeling is saying? How do you know if it's saying, "I could be sisters with her!" or "keep walking"? When the signs are really obvious, it's easy to know. We feel our body relaxing while we talk to a person, or our feet seem to walk away on their own. This is one way our body tells us what it wants us to know.

Your body has a mind all its own. The body's mind is connected with your other mind – the one that thinks your thoughts and knows what you believe. But your body's mind isn't concerned with beliefs or thoughts; it's concerned with how it *feels* and if its systems are running smoothly. It's concerned with survival, but also with thriving. And your body is critically concerned with what you put into it for fuel.

Your thoughts can certainly override what your body is saying. We overrule what our body says all the time by ignoring our gut feelings. We may know, for example, that taking tequila shots now means we're going to hurt the next day, and that we probably shouldn't do it, but it's our *birthday*, so let's ignore that fact - just this once.

It's easy to hear our body when it's yelling at us – the hangover, the huge chin zit, hives, or that chronic condition diagnosis.

We would hear our bodies a lot sooner if we only listened. Paying attention to factors like energy and thirst levels can tell us a lot about a food we just ate. Our moods and emotions can tell us so much about the exercise we do and if we're energizing or pushing ourselves too much.

Your questions about what to eat, when to eat, and how to be as healthy as you can while living with MS all have very specific answers. All you have to do to find them is learn how to listen beyond your thoughts.

Case Study: Me

When I was learning to listen to my body's wisdom, I had to really focus. I had been ignoring my body for a long time, and reconnecting was like making up with an old friend. I started with practicing a body meditation. I listened intently to everything my body was telling me. Every twinge and every flutter was noted.

After a few weeks of this meditation, I sat once again and asked my body what it needed to be healthier. As I asked the question, I was envisioning myself as healthy as possible and what that would look like to me: being fit and at my healthy body weight. As I imagined that outcome, I was hit with something new. I say, "hit" because it really was like a jolt.

"More vegetables," popped into my head, with a stroke of green showing up in my mind's eye.

Seriously? I had to stop and ask myself if that was real. *Did that just happen? Was my mind playing tricks on me?*

I was still relatively new at reading messages from my body, but the answer made sense when I started putting the evidence together. I had been looking at my diet recently and going over my status quo food choices, thinking about how I could level up. Eating more vegetables was clearly how I could make my body healthier. That time, the change wasn't about getting rid of something; it was about adding something in. Admittedly, I wasn't doing an awesome job of getting all my servings of greens each day.

What was born out of that conversation with my body has become a habit for over three years now. I started making green smoothies and have had them almost daily ever since. These smoothies are about 85 percent veggies and 15 percent fruit. Yes, I like how they taste (I'm often asked that question). I even crave them sometimes. When I first started drinking them, I noticed that my energy picked up almost immediately. In fact, whenever I feel run down, a tall glass of salad does the trick every time.

I was able to hear what my body was saying because I was *asking* for its wisdom. Asking your body a question may sound strange, but it works. You can wait for messages from your body for as long as you like, but you'll get them so much faster if you ask a question first.

When was the last time you asked your body what it needed to be healthy? Asking kindly is different from getting mad, believing it doesn't have the answer, becoming frustrated, and going somewhere else for answers. Try being in a quiet setting and asking your body calmly, "What do you need to be healthy?" Do that for a few weeks and see what comes up.

It's fascinating. Promise.

What This Means for You

Chances are, at the conference table of your health team, the head seat has remained empty. The other seats at the table are filled with experts and books and someone's friends' cousin (because they lost weight super fast with a plan you could *totally* do). You're at the table, too, but maybe you're sitting by the water pitcher in case someone needs a refill. Their needs are more important than yours, after all. They're the experts. They know what they're talking about.

I know what your table most likely looks like because mine was filled with the same people for a very long time. Receiving a diagnosis of MS didn't help matters. It just crowded the table with more experts to tell me what to do. I was the water girl, serving all of them in the hope they would tell me the answers. Being passive and doing what I was told was worth it if it helped me achieve a slimmer body and fewer MS symptoms.

Yes, listening to experts with better research than you is helpful. But we also need to leave room at the table for ourselves. You may have been forgetting this, but the new dialogue with your body will confirm that you have a much bigger role than the passive water girl. You have every right to sit at that table, paying full attention.

Our place is at the head of our own table, in the big *Alice In Wonderland* chair.

Setting yourself up as the leader of your health may sound like a bold move, and it is. It's also one of the most important moves you can take.

Making decisions slowly, with large brush strokes at first, will help you ease into it. These are brush strokes that look like eliminating "no-brainer" foods and zeroing in on your hunger. You don't need to go back to school or load up your Kindle with nutrition books. Start with the basics and build from there. If you haven't noticed, this is all about staying the course and making changes for life. More details about how to do that will come sooner than you think.

Let's Go

Once you get used to keeping a food journal, you can amp it up by adding more information. Creating a strong relationship with your body is essential if you want to level up your diet so it's a custom fit to your needs. How do you know if something is or isn't working? You learn how to consult your body.

First up is establishing a routine of checking in with your body. If you're only used to hearing you body when it screams at you, you may need to do this for a few times or for a while before you can hear the calmer notifications. The actual act of checking in with your body is simple: sit quietly and scan over your body to check how it feels. More detailed instructions and a worksheet about how to do a body meditation can be found in Chapter 2 of my first book, *Live Your Life, Not Your Diagnosis.* As you do your body meditation, pay careful attention to your stomach and gut. Do they feel full, bloated, or unhappy in any way? Notice if you're feeling anything in your upper GI tract, like heartburn or pains. Notice the positive side, too. Do you feel like your digestion is running on all cylinders?

Once you've noted how your body is feeling overall, then start to feel your energy levels. Ask yourself these questions:

- *What is my body craving?*
- *What would feel better – going on a walk or going to sleep?*

- *How motivated do I feel when I think about eating healthy food?*
- *How much do I want to eat my favorite junky food?*

These questions are designed to help you see how energized you are and what cravings you have. You may think that craving your favorite junky food is obvious (duh) and will always happen. But when you're eating a clean diet and are in the mode of fostering healthy habits that work for you, cravings for junk mostly disappear and you may crave clean foods instead. Health begets health. This process is a great way to see if you're still eating foods your body doesn't run well on, thus creating cravings for the wrong types of food for you.

Once you've gone through the questions above and have a good idea of how your body and mind are feeling at the moment, ask your body this simple question:

What do I need to feel my best?

Now is when you shut up and listen. The answer may not come to you immediately. It may come but be so subtle that you miss it at first. It will likely come in the form of an idea, or a picture that pops into your head, or a physical feeling. If you feel like taking a nap, that's what your body needs. If you crave something – like vegetables or something fatty – that could be your body telling you that you need more greens or fat in your diet. As you do this more, you will get to know the ways your body best connects with you.

My body connects through ideas that pop into my head. Like *eat more veggies*, or *take a 20-minute power nap*, or even *drink a glass of water*. Sometimes I feel like going for a run right after I ask what my body needs

Twins are known to have special languages and communication between each other that no one else understands. That's how the relationship with your body will be as it strengthens.

Just like with your hunger and emotions, once you get used to checking in with your body, you won't need to sequester yourself in order to listen. Although I still love to meditate and ask my body what it needs, I no longer have to do that to hear my body.

As you get more information directly from your body, compare it with the information in your food journal. You can write in notes about how you feel each day. You can include your mood, any physical sensations, digestion notes, and cravings in your journal. This will allow you to see what you're eating and the real-time effect it has on your body. For example, if you're eating sandwiches every day, but you notice that your brain is foggy, you feel restless, your digestion is off, and you're craving complex carbohydrates, then try going bread free and see how your body reacts.

With this step, you've started to fine-tune your diet to one that works specifically for you.

Future Focus

Life constantly changes. I'm always amused when my clients say that "nothing happened" during the previous week, only to find out during our session, when we dig a little, that four or five important changes happened. They think their lives are stagnant, but they're in a different place than they were even a week ago. I love helping them see how far they've come. As your life changes, it's great to be as on top of it as possible. There are enough surprises out there. If you're like me, you don't want your health to be one of them.

As you strengthen your relationship with your body, you'll become aware of changes much sooner than before. Foods that once fueled you can start to not work as well after a while; a type of exercise that once energized you can become flat and need an upgrade. When you have an illness like MS, symptoms may creep in and drug side effects may come and go.

Our lives constantly change, and our bodies change right along with us.

That's great news, because if you're connecting with your body now, spotting those changes in the future can become effortless. New territory can quickly be traversed and changes put into place without much time lost.

You can give yourself permission at any time to stop feeling pushed around by different advice and advisors. Establishing a routine of connecting with your body now sets you up to feel confident in the changes you make and want to make in your diet and lifestyle. This confidence allows you to take information from teachers and doctors under advisement, but then make an educated decision on your own. You'll no longer feel like someone else knows better than you do about your body. Control over your health will be claimed by its rightful owner: you.

Moving Forward

I love transformation. I think it's amazing that we can take a diagnosis of chronic illness and transform it into an opportunity to be healthier than ever. This ability to transform is an important power we have as human beings.

You have everything you need right now to listen to your body. My past self who was new to this would have a few choice words for me, upon hearing that. It's okay if you do, too. As long as you also have trust. Just like you don't need fancy toys or clothes to make good friends, you also don't need anything outside of yourself to make good friends with your body.

This may seem impossible or frustrating at times. Keep going anyway. You may have trepidation about taking that head seat at the table of your health team when deciding what's best for you. Take a seat anyway and try it out.

You're not cutting out the experts by sitting at the head of your health team table. The opposite is true. You're starting to listen to their advice more thoughtfully. You can try out their advice more deliberately. Instead of throwing things at the wall to see what sticks, you can move through recommendations and really *know* when something works for you. You're no longer wasting time being loyal to strategies that ultimately don't work for you.

How would you rather approach your health? By trying everything blindly, because someone important told you it works? Or by being confident in knowing what strategy you want to try and sensing what is probably snake oil (there's enough snake oil out there to power a small village).

Being able to use what works and leave the rest is a powerful position.

Yes, this process of taking control of your health begins with trust. Trust that your body tells you how it feels. Trust that you can see the patterns in what you're eating and how your body reacts. Trust that you know what's best for your body and that other people, no matter how educated, are only giving you suggestions to try.

Start using that powerful position now and try listening to your body. Give it a week or two and notice what your body tells you. Listen like you're about to hear some juicy gossip. Because that's kind of what it's like. Your body wants to gossip about what you ate yesterday. Does your body have a new love? Or does it want to kick something out immediately because it's creating *way* too much drama?

What you hear can be jaw dropping.

Better than the tabloids.

Chapter 7

Working Out as Simple Math

B y now you may have noticed something that isn't included in this book: research. Generally, books in the self-help genre have loads of research to bolster the author's opinion and give his or her ideas more credibility. I could absolutely have filled this book with research backing up what I discuss and medical terminology detailing how MS works.

But if I did that, this book wouldn't be about you anymore.

Instead, this book would be about MS and how systems in your body can go wrong. It would be about me, and about how the experts I chose to include agree with what I say. It might be interesting information for you, but that's all it would be: information.

In this age of information, we already have more than we can process. We have streams of data coming our way from the internet, the media, and people we talk to each day. We don't even get the information in full detail anymore – only in sound bites or in the form of a title plus the first four sentences of an article.

No, we don't need more information. What we need is to learn how to apply the best of what we already know so we can make all this information *work* for us instead of only being interesting and vaguely useful.

The truth is, I could also find loads of research that backs up the opposite of what I'm saying in this book. Having all of this conflicting information at our fingertips is precisely why people stay confused and do little to improve their health. People stay frozen in place, because it can seem like every step they take has a reported bad consequence.

That is the exact reason I know this book is needed – without research.

Evidence showing whatever you like is out there, I assure you. Looking for more research can be a distraction from you and what you already know. If your doctor plus three other credible sources agree on something, then no more outside consulting is necessary. Close the books and consult yourself instead.

Thinking you need more research when you already have credible sources is a way to say, "I'm not ready yet." If you're not psyched about quitting sugar, you can find a source that says sugar is not that bad for you. If you don't want to change your diet, you can find a source that will tell you that the real answer is something entirely different.

If you find yourself saying, "I don't know," or "What does the research say?" or "I need to find out more," then you're most likely not consulting the crucial person at the head of the table.

Sometimes the reason we don't consult our own bodies is because we know they will tell us how much better it feels without white bread and energy drinks.

What you're learning as you read this book is that, when it comes to knowing if you should eat a cleaner diet, exercise, or adopt other healthy habit, like getting enough sleep, the research and experts have all sorts of opinions. But there's also common ground with what the research and studies say. We're lucky to be in an age when enough studies are being conducted that universal truths are starting to emerge. These universal truths play a big part in how you can lose weight and stay healthy – even with MS.

Many people miss the forest while looking for the trees. I see people every day who are consumed with trying to answer the question "Is gluten bad for me?" while, at the same time, they're going to the drive-thru most days of the week.

In waiting to find and gather *all* the details of what to do to be healthy, people often miss the big picture of how much they can already do.

The common ground of this big picture shows us that:

- sugar and refined carbohydrates aren't great for our bodies,
- ultra-processed foods contain loads of sodium and chemicals that are still mysterious (or that we know make wonderful plastic bags),

- whole ingredients in their original form are good for our bodies
- exercise is good for us.

Our bodies tell us when something is wrong – and also when something is right.

Exercising is just like everything else: you can wait around and scrutinize which exercise is best, or you can just dive in and see for yourself.

Concept: Exercise Is Like Simple Math

Exercise is another area where you can find research in both directions. There's a large body of research that says exercise isn't needed to lose weight – that dropping pounds is all in what you eat, not how you move. Other experts say you do need a baseline of exercise to kick-start your metabolism and lose weight. But, either way you slice it, some form of regular exercise is good for your body.

It's not rocket science. You know you know this.

You're smart. As a logical, intelligent person, you know what can be gained from exercise. There's too much talk in the media about the benefits of working out to ignore it.

But what about when you have MS? Does all of that research still apply to you, or do you need to take it easy?

The amount of research about exercise benefitting people with MS grows each day. Exercise helps with mobility, strength, and flexibility – and with keeping that strength and mobility going into the future. Exercise helps with balance and coordination. Exercise helps us stay cognitively sharp. It's also been suggested that exercise may help slow disease progression entirely. Exercise helps our mood, and helps us lower stress. These are well-known facts about exercise. But these facts take on a whole new meaning when you have MS.

Factors like strength, coordination, and cognitive abilities are all things we want to continue improving well into the future, because these are the very things MS can take from us.

You can lose weight without working out. But your chances of having that independent, exciting future aren't as possible if you're staying on the couch. Living well with a chronic illness means you have to be proactive. Working out is a fantastic way to do that.

Stop waiting for the one, undisputed, absolute, say-it-without-unsaying-it authority to tell you what you should do. Exercise may or may not help directly with losing weight, but it has countless other benefits – some directly relieving for MS symptoms and even easing progression. The decision to work out when you have MS and you want to lose weight is as easy as simple math.

I strongly urge my clients to have some kind of workout program. How intense and what they do is up to them, their level of abilities, and their personalities. For some people, walking around the block or doing 30 minutes of chair stretching every day is fantastic. Others have loved swimming and cycling. The juice isn't in what you choose, though; it's in actually *doing* it.

As humans, we look for the path of least resistance. But sometimes we look for that path so long that we never actually start to walk down it.

So get your cute workout gear on and start. You don't have to be ready to get going. (And there's no research says we can't look cute while we do it.)

Case Study: Sarah

When asked about her workout routine, Sarah gave an answer that most of us can relate to: "I try to walk a few times a week. I hear that's better for the knees than running. I used to walk a lot, but now I guess I don't have so much time for it. I have a big project at work that just started and I have more things in my day than I used to. So I've stopped walking as much."

Then she thought about it more, "I need to get back into it. I was doing really well for a while…"

Then there was a heavy sigh. More stuff to add to her schedule felt overwhelming to Sarah. Even though she knew it was good for her.

Living up to the memory of how much she used to work out was tough. We can torture ourselves with the memory of how "good" we used to be and how we don't stack up anymore.

Sarah knew what we all know – that we should get exercise. But she wasn't in the mode. She'd had a lot of stops and starts. She didn't love the exercise she'd been doing. It felt boring to her. For Sarah, working out was like taking gross-tasting medicine, so she often didn't do it.

If working out feels like something laborious that will take a chunk of time away from your day, it's not going to happen consistently. You will have a lot of stops and starts, like Sarah did, and you'll spend more time remembering how good you used to be instead of actually exercising today.

One thing Sarah had going for her was the desire *to have worked out*. You probably have that desire, too. The desire to have worked out means you like and want the effects of regular exercise, but aren't psyched about actually *doing* the exercise.

That's completely workable.

In the age of podcasts and media and free clubs and (you guessed it) information about working out, finding a workout you like can happen.

That's what Sarah and I did – we found something she could totally do (loving it wasn't necessary yet) and that was located in a place that was easy to for her to get to.

She didn't have time for a class or even always to make the trip to the gym. For her, the answer was high-intensity interval training. It was something she enjoyed that gave her results in as little time as possible.

Instead of trying to find time in her schedule, we worked on how she could make working out a priority. Putting exercise at the top of her priority list helped Sarah go from painfully trying to fit in working out three days a week to easily working out four days a week or more. Taking the pain away from trying to make time changed everything for her.

What This Means for You

Any amount of exercise is good. No matter what it is. That's the good news. You don't have to train for a marathon to get huge positive effects. The effects of exercise come from doing it consistently, not from doing a giant amount at one time. All of the benefits you get from working out will come to you as long as you keep doing it. But if you stop, your body will start to revert back to how it was before you exercised. Muscles will get weaker, flexibility and stamina will decrease. Your energy and fatigue will be negatively affected. Whatever help you get from exercising that contributes to losing weight will be gone as well. We'll talk more about how to stay consistent in the next chapter. For now, just focus on starting – which means making exercise a priority.

When you're thinking about how you can incorporate working out into your busy schedule, keep in mind that this is a life-long commitment. I know that sounds big. It is.

When it comes to losing weight, what we put into our bodies is most important. But I believe working out helps us lose weight as well. Because of what working out does to keep us generally healthy and how it can help our MS, it qualifies as a "no-brainer" category.

You can do anything you like for exercise. As long as your body is moving and you're exerting energy, you're good. Playing with your kids, going out on the water with the kayak club, or going for a walk are all great things to do. And there are many more options. It doesn't matter what you do as long as you do something.

Start by getting to know yourself. Are you a high-intensity kind of person, or do you like calmness? Are you social, or more of a lone wolf? Do you like having fun, or do you prefer being super focused on a goal? Knowing these things about yourself can help shape the type of workout you like and will stick with.

You don't have to go against your grain to get a good workout. In fact, you shouldn't if you want to create a practice you'll stick with. Don't force yourself to do yoga if you think yoga classes are boring. Don't make yourself walk on a treadmill if you loathe working out inside. Don't make yourself join a running group if you would rather get a private running coach and do it on your own time. This is the 21st century. You can find something to enjoy.

You may also change your workout as time goes on – in fact, it's likely that you will. I'm always changing things around to keep my interest. I make it a priority to find something that works, and I constantly ask myself how I can make working out better. If you keep asking yourself the same thing, you will find your sweet spot for working out, too – over and over again.

Let's Go

What are you doing for exercise these days? Think about the past few weeks, but don't go back any farther than that. The "I used to" answer doesn't help you.

How many times a week are you exercising? How much exercise?

Working out six times a week for an hour may sound like the right answer for you, but it may not be the right answer if it means you're beat for the rest of the day. When it comes to exercise, doing it smarter, not harder, is the key.

First, take a moment to decide if you want to workout. Then ask yourself why or why not. Make sure your answer is solid. Consider it information to help you get the exercise your body needs.

If you're not working out at all right now, be curious about why. Do you feel like there's no time after you do everything for everyone else? Do you simply not want to make time? If the answer is that you don't want to make the time, ask yourself why you don't want to. Notice if you're happy with your answer.

Reconnect with why you *do* want to work out. This reason is super important, because even with the best plans there will be days you don't want to exercise. For example, a big reason why I work out is that it keeps me mentally sharp. That's a big yes for me, and connecting with that reason will get me going even when it's freezing outside.

When you have an established workout routine, determine if what you're doing is harder than it needs to be. It's important to make this distinction between hard enough and too hard, because pushing your body too hard will catch up with you. You don't have to go to crazy lengths for exercise to be beneficial. That's certainly not the way to become a person who regularly works out.

On the days you do work out, how does your body feel? You may feel spent at first, but working out should ultimately energize you. If you're going full-out for an hour every morning, but then feel like you can't do anything else for the rest of the day, you're doing too much.

Keep a log of what your workout is and how you feel during the day. If you vary your workouts, you may find that you feel differently, depending on what you do and when and how much. Cardio may zap you, but doing weights may make you feel good for the rest of the day. By looking at how working out affects you, you can also find how to get the most benefits.

My cardio is a first-thing-in-the-morning deal. I happen to like running and high-intensity interval training, but if I don't get it done in the morning, it's probably not going to happen. But working out with weights at the gym is fine to do at the end of my day. They're two different types of workouts, and I know when I perform best during and after each one.

This is the type of information we get from listening to our bodies. On the days you decide to workout, write down what and how much you do. Then ask yourself the following questions at the end of the day:

- *Did I feel energized when I worked out, or did I feel like I had to pull myself along?*
- *Do I feel like I did too much or just enough?*
- *How did I feel right after the workout?*
- *How did I feel a few hours after that?*
- *Did I get more or less done in my day than I usually do?*

Answering these questions will help you assess whether that workout was right for you.

Ask your body if what you did worked. Your body will know. Listen for the answer. If the answer is that you need to slow down, listen and act accordingly. Our energy has peaks and valleys, too. Tapping into how you're physically feeling allows you to work with the flow instead of against it. Don't be discouraged if you did more the previous week and feel you need to slow down for a bit this week. You're creating habits for life. Slowing down for a bit because your body asks you to will help you stay consistent in the long term. Rest is an important part of a workout routine and necessary to help you do more in the long run.

Future Focus

When you're in the mode of exercising consistently, the effects have a ripple effect on the future you. Exercise may or may not be your key to losing weight, but it can be the key to having that independent future you crave.

Think again about what you most want in your future. You probably want independence. Maybe you want to travel to unique places, have a long career, and have financial stability. My hunch is that happiness plays a big part in your future visions as well. All of those things can be positively affected by starting a consistent workout practice now that you can continue for life.

When you start really diving into what makes working out a priority for you, and how you can do it consistently, the bumps in the road won't be such a problem. There will be times when working out *should* take a back seat – like if you have an injury or a flare up of MS, for example. There are weeks that taking a break from working out will be a good option for you, and your body can tell you when that is.

When you think of yourself as "someone who works out," you can take a week or so off and then you'll get right back into it again. Those hiccups won't be so frustrating if you know that, when it comes to a lifetime of working out, a week of down time is not a big deal.

Start Where You Are Now

Finding your workout zone may seem tough at times. Especially if you're currently not doing much to speak of. Take it a step at a time. You don't need to psych yourself out about exercise.

It can help to pay attention to the specifics about what you're doing, because then you have some data to work with. Start slowly. Do the minimum amount that you can do each week, and stick with that at first. That may mean you exercise once a week, or it may mean three times a week. Build on it when you can, but get used to being a person who consistently works out – do that by starting with something you can easily stick with.

Play around with what you choose to do for exercise. That's how you'll find something you love to do – and something you will keep doing.

Maybe your minimum is walking three times a week for 20 minutes, but you realize you hate walking on a treadmill. You can keep that three times a week minimum, but move your walks outside. Or you can ditch walking entirely and give that spin class a try. If you have your minimum you'll do each week, you can play within that parameter to find what you love. The simple math is to find the minimum and build on that without letting it drop.

Most of all, give yourself credit for what you do.

There's not much I can tell you that you don't already know about why we should workout consistently. What I *can* help you with is making sure it happens.

Just like being curious about what you're eating, be curious about what you're doing for exercise now. Do you like it? Do you believe you can like it? Really taking the time to think about not only what you do to work out, but knowing what you believe about it can make or break your habit.

If you believe exercise has to suck in order to work, it will. But it really doesn't have to be that way.

Encourage yourself. Be a friend who exercises with you as a companion, instead of a screaming trainer berating you from the sidelines.

With every workout, know that you're building the future you crave.

Nurture yourself and you will find workouts that nurture you.

⌒ ⌒ ⌒

Do you want to work out more, but:

- Think there's no way it will fit into your busy schedule?
- Working out zaps your energy?
- Don't know how much is enough and worry about doing too little or too much?

Listen to the free downloadable class from me. Visit: **www.AndreaHansonCoaching.com/Learnmore.**

Chapter 8

When You're Consistently Inconsistent

We can all relate to the concept of inconsistency. We start a new routine with excitement – and then it fizzles. It's not that we don't believe in the changes we want so badly to make. But the belief that we can make them a normal everyday practice isn't always there.

Fizzling out can happen when we start anything – for example, working out, wanting to quit gluten, or wanting to stop cursing (full disclosure: I've never actually tried to stop cursing, but I hear it's difficult). Think about a big change you've made recently. My bet is that you can track its progress from charging out of the gate to the finish line that came way sooner than you expected.

Why do we put ourselves through this every time we want to create a new habit? Why do we keep believing that "it's different this time," when it rarely is?

Some people think MS makes them resistant to slacking off when it comes to their health, and then are disappointed when they approach exercise the way they always have. I've thought that as well. I thought having MS meant I'd "get serious" about my health. Like the disease itself would change how I approached my health. I was sorely disappointed when I realized that having this disease doesn't automatically make me more invested in my health. The truth is that there are many people with MS who don't want to change their health at all. MS doesn't decide anything for you. You're the one who makes the decision to create life-long change.

If you're putting the onus on MS to make a change for you, stop it. It's not the MS that has the power to make you change. It's you.

◠ ◡ ◠

Why is it that when there's a perfectly logical change you want to make, your effort seems to fizzle? Maybe not immediately, but at some point. Think back over the past year. What's your batting average with consistently keeping up new routines?

To help you find that answer, let's look first at what *consistency* means. Most would say it means *sticking to it* – doing the same thing over and over again. That's one aspect of consistency, but there's a larger piece that often gets overlooked.

The *idea* of being a consistent person happens before you *act* consistently. Many people who fizzle out are missing this larger piece of being successful. In Chapter 7, I said people often don't exercise because they aren't seeing the forest for the trees. They're so focused on the trees, the action of creating a new habit (and the frustration that comes with not keeping said habit), that they miss the forest, the macro understanding that they need to believe they're a person who consistently takes action. The same concept applies to consistency. Focusing on the forest is having thoughts like *I work out consistently. I am always interested in being healthy. I am a healthy person.* When you have an overarching belief that you will do it, the details of the action become easier.

Being consistent is different from creating a habit. Habit is the action. Consistency is a frame of mind.

When you adopt the belief that you are a consistent person, the action piece will fall into place much more easily.

Concept: Consistency is a State of Mind

What comes to mind when you imagine yourself as being someone who consistently eats what your body needs? When I was at my heaviest weight, I would think about what kind of a person I would be when I was thinner and healthier. I imagined being steadfast in what I would put into my body. I imagined that I would work out all the time, no question. I imagined that I would never mess around with my health. *How could I? I have MS now and need to lose the weight for real this time.* I remember throwing that logic to myself.

For me, consistency in my health meant that I would waiver very little from my healthy routine. I now know that believing

I had to have a near perfect record was one of the reasons I felt like I failed all the time at making the changes I knew would be good for me.

Consistency isn't a straight line to done. It doesn't mean having only a few "cheat days" and otherwise being on point the rest of the time. When you're consistent, there are still stops and starts. There are still times when you feel like it's easy and other times it's so hard you don't think you'll make it.

Gaining weight, eating a hamburger with all the fixin's, not working out for a week – these can all be examples of being consistent in your weight loss. Counterintuitive? Not really.

When you have the mindset that you are a consistent person when it comes to your health, things like gaining weight are par for the course. Here's why: when you're a consistent person and you gain weight, instead of digging into that pint of ice cream while you contemplate your failure, you figure out why you got tripped up and thus reduce the chance that it will happen again.

When you believe that you're consistent in your health, you understand that nothing has gone wrong. Even if there's a month of lackluster workouts – or no workouts – and cheese plates after every meal, if you think of yourself as a consistent person in your efforts to be healthy you can use the experience to learn more about how you can stay healthy for life. And then getting back to your routine is not hard at all. Because when you have a mindset that you're a consistent person, you know that you haven't failed. You've simply experienced the ebb and flow of getting healthy.

Case Study: Billy

Billy had arrived at a point of utter frustration. "I can't do this anymore," he said. "I keep gaining weight. This obviously isn't working. I don't know what else to do."

He was focusing less and less on the changes he had previously decided to make – changes like training for a 5K he had signed up to do in a month and not eating sugar. The numbers on the scale were crushing him, leading him to believe he was failing miserably.

"Look, there's no point in trying to be good," he said about sticking to the changes. "I obviously don't want to change, or I would have done it already."

Billy had shut down. The week before we spoke he had gone on a binge-fest. He let his actions be the evidence he needed to prove to himself that he would never lose weight. He had temporarily lost the belief that he was a person who was interested in his health. He believed, instead, that he obviously wasn't interested in health – because he hadn't been doing what he wanted to do.

I wasn't buying that logic, because he was missing a crucial point. There's a difference between believing that our past performance shows us who we are as a person, and believing that our performance teaches us how to become better – even if our performance comes with a side of fries.

For Billy, the switch in thinking came when he realized that his past week was not a failure. He came to understand that his "failure" was loaded with opportunities to discover what was holding him back.

We talked about what he was making the scale mean and how that led him to feel like a disappointment. When he felt like a failure, it was only natural that he "failed" at eating well.

His perspective came into focus when he realized that he had never stopped believing that he was interested in health. It was that belief that pulled him back on course. If he had thought instead that he'd fallen off the wagon and so had to start over again, then getting back into a healthy routine would have been much harder.

What This Means for You

From a very young age, we believe that the proof lies in the evidence. But what we're not taught is that we can find evidence to prove anything we like. Billy was using the evidence eating crappy food to prove he would never lose weight. It's a logical argument, from a certain perspective. If you eat too much junk food, you will gain weight.

But that's not all the evidence that was available to him. It was just the evidence he decided to use. Billy could have chosen to see eating junk food as evidence that he still had thoughts that were causing him to eat it. It was his call whether to see the junk food as evidence of a flag signaling another path to explore, or as evidence of a dead end. His belief that he was a consistently healthy person helped him choose the junk food to be an opportunity, not a failure.

We can choose anything we like and use it as evidence. The question is: are you choosing good evidence that helps you or bad evidence that demotivates you?

You may not see this as a choice. You may see your behavior as meaning only one thing – whether you're staying consistent with your new habits or you're not. But that black and white thinking isn't helpful for life-long changes. Life is not all or nothing, and neither is the process of losing weight and being healthy.

When it comes to your weight loss, which evidence are you choosing?

Finding evidence is easier than you think. Even if you feel completely frustrated, like Billy did at first, you can search for and find helpful evidence to keep you going. And I mean real evidence, not pretense.

Knowing how to spot it when you're using bad evidence can stop the feelings of failure. And as you practice using good evidence, that skill will only grow and show you how far you've come and how easy it can be to stay on track.

Keeping the overall belief that you're consistently healthy becomes easier, too.

Let's Go

Focusing on bad evidence keeps you from being consistent.

Evidence is bad when it proves something that makes you feel... well... bad. For example – using the fact you ate cake as evidence to prove that you'll never lose weight. Or using the fact that you skipped your Pilates class to finish the reality TV show as evidence that you can't get into the habit of working out. Bad evidence serves to beat us down and can keep us from believing that health is in our grasp. Understanding the difference between good and bad evidence and which type you're using is essential when you want to create a consistently healthy mindset.

To understand the evidence, understand what you want to prove to begin with: get clear about your hypothesis. Knowing what you're trying to prove points toward the type of evidence you're looking for.

Let's look at a few hypotheses that you already have. Ask yourself this question: *What do I think about losing weight?*

List the first three things that come to mind. For example, you may think that losing weight is hard. You may think it will take a long time or a lot of hard work to get to your natural weight. A common hypothesis is that it's easier to gain weight than to lose it.

Each of those thoughts is a hypothesis that you will naturally look for evidence to prove.

Take, for example, the hypothesis that it's easier to gain weight than to lose it. If that were your hypothesis, your brain would go to task looking for all the reasons why that's right. The brain naturally looks for evidence to prove what we're thinking. It makes no sense to believe something that we know is wrong, so our brains have a marked interest to make sure what we believe is right.

Your brain will look for all sorts of evidence to prove that it's easier to gain weight than to lose it. The evidence you'll pick out may be about how easy it is to eat more than one brownie, or how slowly you think the numbers on the scale are moving down. You may find evidence in how hard it is to stay motivated or how these jeans are maybe fitting more snugly than the last time you wore them.

You can nit-pick as much as you like when looking for evidence to prove that gaining weight is easier than losing it. But how does your evidence make you feel? My guess is, not awesome. That's how you know you're looking for bad evidence.

What if, instead, your hypothesis was *losing weight is easy?* What if you went to task looking for evidence to prove that right? You'd be able to prove that hypothesis as well, because evidence always exists. It's a matter of what we're purposefully looking for. You can purposefully look for evidence and find: your body feels good, you worked out yesterday, maybe you've gone down a size, or you skipped dessert at lunch without thinking twice. There is all sorts of evidence to prove that losing weight is easy. And how do you feel when you believe losing weight is easy? I know it feels awesome, because I've done that work myself.

To find your hypothesis, ask yourself these questions:

- *What do I think about losing weight?*
- *What do I think about my body?*
- *What do I think about working out?*
- *What do I think about my MS?*

List the first three answers you have to each one of these questions. Then look at the evidence you have to prove each one. How does the evidence make you feel? Are you looking for evidence to support a positive or a negative hypothesis?

The biggest question here is: *Is this hypothesis something I want to believe?* If not, put your brain to task proving something better.

Both the hypothesis and the evidence are your choices.

Future Focus

Imagine that you believe, with all your heart, the thought *I'm consistent with my health*. What would 20 years of believing that thought look like?

When you have a consistent mindset, you won't fall into not-so-healthy routines for very long. Maybe it will last a month at the most. Be even if those not-so-healthy routines last longer, you will always return to a health-driven path. That's because you'll never lose your identity as someone who's healthy. Even as you're chewing on candy corn, you will know health is a path that you can get back on.

If you think you're having a bad day, you will know it's just one day out of your entire life. That broad perspective makes getting back into a healthy routine that you know works for you much easier than if you think you need to start all over again.

When you're consistent with your health over a long period of time, you're in a position to tweak your plan much more easily. When you're consistent with your health, you can see very quickly how changes affect you. You can also see what you need more clearly. When you're consistently coloring with green, you notice very quickly when you switch to red. But if you're consistently coloring with all different colors, the red will slip by for a longer time before you notice it.

Before you have consistent actions, you must have a consistent mindset. When you focus on keeping the belief that you're a consistently healthy person, staying healthy becomes more like an identity than an option. More than anything, keeping a consistent frame of mind around being healthy will set you up for the future you want to have.

Start Where You Are Now

There's a reason why "consistency is key" is a cliché. Consistency determines a large chunk of your health. But it doesn't start with the actions – it starts with what you believe.

Staying consistent with actions can sometimes feel like swimming upstream. We can start with too many changes at once, and then we watch them fall like dominos when we see that our actions aren't consistent.

But I promise you're never starting at square one, even though it may feel like it each time you start a new routine.

Start with one or two changes at a time – and in completely different categories. For example, change something about how you eat, like cutting out a "no-brainer" food, and then also change the number of days you work out. Those changes don't overlap – they're actions around different aspects of health – so you're less likely to confuse the messages your body gives you in response. When you're consistent with those changes for a month, then you can change something else. As you practice this methodical way of making changes by focusing on a consistent mindset and listening to your body's messages, tweaks to your lifestyle will become more fluid.

As you stay consistent, you will see more evidence that what you're doing is working, like, for example, you'll see weight loss and that you're losing the taste for super sweet food. Proof for a hypothesis that feels good will become much easier to find. Once you start this cycle, it will seem to flow onward on its own.

You may not feel like you've been very consistent with your weight loss or with eating healthy. Part of that may be from simply being confused about where to start.

That feeling of inconsistency can end right now.

Start with a focus on the belief that you're interested in being consistently healthy. Or maybe there's another belief akin to that one that works better for you. Find one that hits the spot, and be consistent in your belief.

That's how you get a lifetime membership to being healthy.

Chapter 9

How to Stay Motivated

Discovering what makes you lose weight so you can have the future you crave is why you picked up this book. You've learned many things already about where to start, the big changes you can make right now, and how to keep health as a consistent mindset and lifestyle. Making those changes and moving forward with a consistent plan is fantastic.

Upon learning this, you may have an initial burst of excitement. You may be thinking, *I know what to do! I know how to do this! I know I can make big changes that create big shifts in my health.* And you're right. You can start now. In fact, I hope you have.

Inspiration is something that comes from factors largely outside yourself – from a book or a personal story, for example. However, being inspired to make changes can only help you go so far, because inspiration is a finite resource. Inspiration runs out, and if there isn't anything around to inspire you further, the spark can fizzle.

Motivation, however, is a driving force within us that is a renewable resource. Before we can create a mindset that works, before we take action, and certainly before we can make actions consistent, we must be motivated. Once we locate and tap into that motivation, renewing it doesn't depend on anything outside of us.

If we're not motivated to do something, it won't get done. Our actions will fade because we have to *want* to make the change. We can rely on inspiration and tactics to try and make changes in our health, but if we lack the sheer motivation to change, we won't get far at all.

If you don't have motivation, what changes you do implement can feel like an uphill battle. Taking action is much harder if, in your heart, you don't really want to do it. Taking action can be grueling if you're doing it because someone is "making you" or "wants you to" do it. That's why it can sometimes feel so hard to lose weight – when we're doing it in ways other people tell us to do. It may be a logical assumption that *of course* you want to lose weight – but that's not motivation. And this is a big part of why this weight loss thing can be confusing.

Concept: Creating Motivation

Motivation is the very first thing to consider when making changes. Being motivated means we *want* to do something. Before I have my clients make any changes at all, I ask them, "Do you *want* to do this?" Their answer to that question is everything.

It doesn't matter how squeaky-clean your mindset is, a lack of motivation will trump it every time. You can believe something is the right thing to do – and you can even believe what we talked about in Chapter 8, that you're a consistently healthy person – but none of those thoughts matter if you don't *want* to make a change.

Simply put, if you don't *want* to do something, you won't do it for long.

The good news is that you're in total control of your mindset and, thus, in control of feeling motivated and wanting to do something.

So, how do you get that motivation?

There's a growing body of research that's centered on video games and how to duplicate the extreme motivation that gamers have for gaming and apply it to real life. Jane McGonigal, video game designer, researcher, and author of *Reality Is Broken: Why Games Make Us Better And How They Can Change the World*, writes about the impressive motivation gamers have when they spend hours solving often very difficult games. To spend that much time, gamers must have a lot of motivation to stay connected, even when it looks like all is lost. What McGonigal and other video game creators and researchers in the positive psychology field are finding out is that there are quite a few factors that effect motivation. I teach two of these factors regularly because they can be a superhighway to staying motivated.

The first one is giving yourself rewards. Rewards are extremely important if you want to keep the motivation going. I'm not talking about things like a mani-pedi or a massage. Those kinds of rewards are not what will keep you going. We can give ourselves those types of rewards anytime, and so withholding them for lack of performance creates a nasty cycle.

The reward that works the best is simple acknowledgement. Literally the high fives. This works for a few reasons. One is that we're giving ourselves validation, and validation feels good. We often seek it from other people, but it means the most when we get real validation from ourselves. Every time you do something toward staying healthy, stop and notice what you're doing. Every time you find that good evidence, take a moment and bring your attention to it. These validations can serve as mile markers that keep you wanting more of the same.

The second factor that can fuel motivation is the belief that whatever you're doing can be accomplished. Believing something can be done is so often overlooked. People believe they can try, they believe other people can do it, but the absolute belief that it can be done by them is often lacking. I go a step further with my clients and help them believe that it's already done – then they just have to do the work. When you believe like this, the motivation to do the work is easy.

Motivation is instantly created when you connect with the belief that you can accomplish anything you try. For example, believing that losing the weight is a sure thing, that becoming healthy is absolutely possible, that being independent well into the future has already been decided. When you adopt this outlook, the motivation flows.

On the contrary, if you don't believe weight loss is possible, you probably won't see great results. Or you'll lose weight while complaining the whole time. I've been there – this is when I lost a ton of weight and then gained it all back and more. I bitched and moaned the whole time (I'm sure I was fantastic to be around).

Motivation will not be there if you don't think something is possible. Why would you want to do something that isn't possible? You won't.

Case Study: Kelly

Kelly had already been through a few cycles of gaining and losing weight before she started working with me. She knew the stress of that cycle wasn't good for her body and she had new motivation to stop it because she had been diagnosed with MS just a few months earlier.

She started by telling me her story. "So I've tried this one diet, and it was great. I felt awesome and lost a ton of weight."

"Great," I said, "So why did you sign up for coaching?"

"Well, I didn't stick with that diet. I just kind of stopped doing it. It was hard, and I like to go out with friends and stuff, you know? I couldn't really do that on this diet."

Kelly thought she was super motivated to lose weight. She knew how good her body felt on that specific diet, so she knew there were components of it that really worked for her. Staying on the diet for a while had even helped her lose weight. If everything was working for her body so well, why didn't she stay on that diet forever?

Because she didn't want to.

Sure, she was motivated to lose weight, but when we drilled down to her taking the steps to follow the actual diet, it became clear that she didn't want to do it. So she didn't.

And she did what most of us do after a "failed" diet – she blamed herself for not following through, and got mad at her lack of willpower.

She beat herself up.

"Do you believe that this diet is sustainable for you?" I asked her after she recounted what happened.

"No. It was hard and it got in the way of my life."

There was one huge factor of her motivation that was missing: she didn't believe she could do it. So it makes sense that she stopped doing it. Why would she keep doing something that was so hard if she didn't believe she would do it sustainably? She had all sorts of evidence showing her that she couldn't stay on that diet.

She had done the same thing before with other diets. She would get sold on the extreme results that each diet "could" give her. But her stance was the same each time: she didn't actually believe she could pull it off.

The first thing we looked at was what she did want to do. Yes, she did want to lose weight, but there was a whole other level of action that she needed to be motivated to do, and she wasn't. When we stopped working on following strict diets and started to find a custom diet for her, Kelly found her motivation again. When she saw the direct relationship between specific foods and how she felt, it was much easier for her to find that enthusiasm and keep up her motivation.

When she was following other diets, even though she felt fantastic, it was hard to stay with them because, although she was inspired and motivated to lose weight, her motivation to stick with an intense diet fell short.

What This Means for You

There are quite a few reasons it's hard to stick with a diet. Most diets will help you lose weight if you do everything they say. You can cut out five different food groups and probably drop 30 pounds in a month. That's technically working, right? I have talked to plenty of people – and this goes for me, too – who have been on diets that worked, but they don't stick with it and a major reason was the lack of motivation.

Sometimes lacking the motivation to stick with a diet is your body saying "no." (More on this in Chapter 11.)

You can build your motivation by starting with what you (and your body) actually want to do.

Some people protest here because they think that what they actually want is to sit on the sofa spraying squirt cheese directly in their mouths while watching trashy TV every day.

I always call their bluff – and I'll call yours, too, if you think you want that.

Ask yourself, really, what you want to do to get healthy.

How do you want to feel? What do you want working out to be like? Fun? Hanging out with friends? Goal-oriented, so the evidence that feels good piles up?

What do you want your diet to be like? Easy? Fast? Creative?

Consider what you want first, then start to build your changes around that.

When you start with what you want, motivation is created. As you explore what you want and then, little by little, create that custom plan, you will shift into the belief that it can, in fact, be done. That's how you create the motivation you need and make it dependent on nothing other than you.

Let's Go

Just as validation can create motivation, withholding validating can snatch that motivation away faster than you can say "pie." Withholding validation can happen more often than we realize.

Sometimes we get the little personal trainer in our minds who's making sure we work hard and stay on point. But often that little voice says things like, *You're not working hard enough* or – a favorite of the voice in my head – *You have to do more before it counts.*

We don't give ourselves enough credit for what we do. Maybe we think giving credit will make us stop working. Maybe it will make us not go as hard as we can. One of the biggest shifts for me came when I told that little voice in my head to go away. I did it nicely, because it was only trying to help. But I told the little trainer in my head, in no uncertain terms, that it was not helping one bit.

Not giving ourselves credit for what we actually have done on our way to a lifestyle change is an interesting paradox. Here's something we really, really want – losing weight. But we don't give ourselves credit for all we've done toward accomplishing it. Chances are, you're doing way more than you think you are, but you aren't letting yourself have the satisfaction of acknowledging that you're working hard.

Here's how you can change that: find your evidence. Write down everything you're currently doing to get healthy or that you've tried ˜ do in the past. For example, you can list how often you worked ˖ you've tried to change in your diet, if you've stopped smoking. (Caveat: if you're smoking cigarettes, it's time to quit. It's especially bad for your MS and can escalate problems quickly. No messing around here.)

Create a list – it doesn't matter if what you did worked or not. Show yourself everything you've done in the past year.

Look at your list and check off everything that you truly wanted to do. As always, get super honest with yourself. You may have wanted the results, but did you really want to do all of that?

Now create a different list. This list is of what you *want*. Answer these questions to create your list:

- *What do I want for my body?*
- *What do I want for my future?*
- *What do I want financially, as well?* (Because it's related.)

Look at this list and check off everything you have already. Be honest. Some of it you may have and some you may not. That's ok.

Visualize yourself having everything on your list. *Hold that feeling in your body.*

That is what motivation feels like.

Future Focus

Knowing what you want is essential. We can take it for granted that we know what we want, but then why do we do so many things we don't want to do? If your answer is, "Because we're grown-ups and that's just what we have to do," I call B.S. on that.

Think of that future self you've been creating. When you envision your future self as healthy and at a natural weight, are you also envisioning being and doing all sorts of things that future you doesn't want to do? My hunch is no.

Your future self is awesome because you'll get there by being motivated to make those changes. That is not a person who got where she will be by kicking and screaming. You get there by knowing what you want, knowing what works, and having true motivation and desire to get there.

Motivation can make or break any habit, routine, or choice. If you're not motivated to do something, it won't happen, and it certainly won't become a choice you stick with for the long haul.

My bet is that you want consistency. You want motivation. And you probably want losing weight to be easier than it has been in the past. It all starts with *wanting* to do something every step of the way.

Knowing what you want to do – and why – will carry you far into the future.

It may seem ludicrous to *want* to give up sugar or processed foods or to want to start working out on the regular, but call your own bluff. Getting honest with what you really do want is how your healthy, svelte, independent future is created.

Start With Where You Are Now

I'm not saying that your motivation will be at warp speed all the time if you "just believe." That's not true – and it's annoying. What I am saying is that being motivated is 100 percent your call.

Your motivation will wax and wane. Sometimes it will be easy to get your shoes on and go to the gym. Other times it will feel like pulling teeth. But understanding more about your motivation and what goes into it makes it easier to pull yourself up, even if your first thought is "I don't wanna."

Start by giving yourself those high fives. Seriously. Every time you take a step toward health, give yourself validation. Choosing to not eat dessert, even though everyone at the table is – high five. Choosing to go for a walk around the block – high five. Choosing to finish this book and do all the exercises – high five *and* a low five.

Giving that credit is important, because what we tend to focus on is that we're missing out on what everyone else can eat, that we're not really walking that far, and that this book alone can't *make* you do anything. Chances are, you've been pelting yourself with downers for a long time.

Then focus on what you believe can happen. You may also need to start small here, and that's completely okay. This is a practice, and the skills are the same whether you practice them on believing you can change the world or believing you can read to the end of this sentence.

What do you believe will happen with your health? Do you believe you can lose 50 pounds? Do you believe you can say "no" to the next cookie that's offered to you? Start looking at what you believe for sure now, and then keep building from there.

Staying motivated doesn't have to be rocket science – in fact, it's way better if it's not. Keep it simple and start with where you are now. When you get a good feel for what you want and what you believe, building from there is be easier.

You're not building an algorithm. You're getting honest and serious with yourself. It may feel like a test, but don't worry – no one has to see your answers if you don't want them to.

Chapter 10

Mind Your Power

When making a change, we often start by focusing on the actions we need to take. Seems logical, right? A saying attributed to Mahatma Gandhi reads, "Be the change that you wish to see in the world." If you want a change in your world, you can do something yourself to make it happen. And sometimes the best thing you can do is change your thinking.

I often talk with people with MS who want to change their diet. Their first question is usually, "What should I do?" They're looking to me to suggest a specific diet or to teach them how to be accountable for their actions. It's exciting when the people I talk with want to be proactive about their health. However, if their focus is only on what to do and how to do it, they miss out on a major player in this game of change: what they think. Gandhi spoke about resisting passively and creating peace, but he also knew that what we think creates how we behave.

Thoughts come first. We have thoughts before every emotion we have, every action we take, and every result we see in our life.

In Chapter 5, we looked at feelings and the crucial role they play in losing weight. We saw that the real reason we do anything is to feel better or to stop feeling bad. If we're feeling disheartened, it's much harder be motivated to pay attention to our health. If we're feeling empowered and successful, staying the path and saying "no" to our favorite ice cream is much easier. How we think drives how we feel. How we feel drives our actions.

Which means that if what you think isn't supportive of the action you want to take, that action won't last for long. How can we stop eating bread if we think that it probably doesn't really matter if we eat it? How can we make working out a priority if we think that we won't be able to get into shape? How can we take action to lose weight if we think that we have to take care of our sick friend before we can focus on ourselves?

Throughout this book, we've been touching on how our thoughts create our actions. I've posed questions to ask you about what you really want, whether your mindset is helping you stay consistent, and why you eat (especially when you snack or simply pop something in your mouth). What you've been doing is helping you gain an understanding of what you *believe*. Thoughts are beliefs in their most simplified form.

Wanting someone to "just tell me what to do" is a common desire when it comes to getting healthy, especially if your life has been rocked with a diagnosis. You may feel powerless and unqualified as you assess your current situation. But if you take a deeper dive into thought awareness, you'll see that a complete deferral to someone else's thoughts does not serve you.

What you think is at the hub of everything in your life. Being *aware* of what you think is crucial, especially if you're considering taking advice from others.

Concept: Being the Curious Witness

A page out of all of our childhoods tells the story of our parents, or another authority figure, looking down on us and demanding an answer to that infamous trick question, "What were you thinking?!"

When I was posed that question after getting caught toilet papering the pink adobe house at the top of the hill, I said what most of us say: "I don't know." *We thought it would be fun. We thought it would be hilarious. We thought it would go down as middle school legend* (and it was for at least a week). But I kept those answers to myself. I instead succumbed to the pressure and said, "I don't know what I was thinking."

I totally missed the point. I *did* know exactly what I had been thinking. But I brushed off what I knew because saying what I really thought would have earned me at least another week of being grounded.

Time has passed since we told our moms, "I don't know why I did that" and something was taken away in order to teach us responsibility.

But often we're still stuck in that mode.

Only now we have thoughts like, *I don't know what to eat. I need someone to tell me what to eat and make me responsible.* We've become so accustomed to believing that we don't know what we're thinking that, even if we have an idea of our thoughts, we brush it aside as unhelpful.

Nothing could be further from the truth.

Everything you think is helpful to you. Getting in touch with your mind and understanding how your thoughts flow through to the actions you take is one of the most helpful things you can do.

Chances are, you're used to brushing off many of your thoughts as unhelpful. For example, you may have had a whisper of *I can't do this,* but put it aside as not beneficial to your cause of losing weight. But in order to open the door to understanding what you're thinking at any given time so you can address the thoughts that aren't serving you, you'll need to listen to your mind without judgment.

If you stopped to critique yourself every time you took a step, you wouldn't get very far in a race. Stopping to critique each thought won't get you very far in understanding what thoughts are running through your head, either.

Begin by simply getting curious.

Curiosity is the perfect way to approach our minds. We're not judging or dismissing anything. We're inviting something forward so we can take another look. This is a calm, friendly way to find out about what's happening in our heads. When we find that we're thinking something detrimental to our cause (which I promise we all do), staying in the energy of acceptance is the perfect place to be as we begin to manage that thought.

When you're planning your weight loss, understanding how to manage your own mind is the ultimate skill.

Case Study: Eva

A student in one of my workshops was frustrated as she told me how she couldn't stick with any diet. She very much wanted to, and I believe that her motivation was firmly in place, but she didn't think she had the willpower to do it.

"How do I stop myself from grabbing chips when I go grocery shopping for detergent?"

This is a common question that I've heard from more than one person, including myself.

"What do you expect to happen when you go shopping?" I asked. "Do you expect to stick with the list or do you expect you'll grab some chips?"

She didn't answer, but she started nodding her head. She got it. She was expecting to grab the chips.

What she hadn't realized was that by focusing on the *problem* of grabbing the chips when she grocery shopped, she was playing that thought over and over in her head. *It's a problem that I'm going to grab the chips.*

There's no mystery that when we're focused and thinking constantly about unwanted behavior, we end up doing that unwanted behavior.

It would be really helpful for Eva to look more closely at what she was thinking about those chips. Why did she feel like she needed them? What thoughts threatened to pop into her head when she didn't grab them? What thoughts was she avoiding by focusing on the chips?

By understanding the deeper meaning we're attaching to "cheat" food, we can begin to understand exactly why we reach for it – and then it's much easier to stop.

What This Means for You

Here are several common and yet completely unhelpful thoughts that often flow through our minds:

- *I have no choice.*
- *I can't help it.*
- *I don't know.*
- *It's not enough.*
- *It isn't happening fast enough.*
- *I don't have the willpower.*
- *This should be easier.*
- *I don't know how to do this.*

The good news is you're not alone if any number of these thoughts swirl in your head. We all have fearful thoughts akin to these. The bad news is, they can stop productivity in its tracks. Quite often these thoughts are simply accepted as facts. But they're not facts and they're not the bottom line. There are deeper, more helpful thoughts behind each thought on that list, if we only inquire. But we tend to stop at thoughts like those and let them wreak their havoc.

Understanding our own mindsets is not a new concept. Although many people practice awareness, often they don't go deep enough into what they're thinking to get to the core of what drives their actions. This is where you can apply your curiosity and ask the crucial questions that will allow you to go deeper into your thinking.

The deeper your understanding is of what you're thinking, the deeper your understanding is of what drives you. When you have that deep understanding of why you're resistant to doing some things and drawn to doing others, you're able to make changes with far more velocity.

The power of thoughts can often be dismissed as fluff. But that dismissal leaves a powerful tool behind.

The first proof of real change isn't doing it, it's believing in it. You can will yourself into some impressive changes, but unless what you truly think is supportive of what you're doing, your actions will fizzle when you either deliberately give up, or when you feel like you're sabotaging yourself.

Looking more deeply at your thoughts is your chance to dig your teeth into something that will stick to your bones as you make changes. Going deeper into your thoughts may be a new practice for you, but it must be done if you want to be in line with your health for life.

Let's Go

If you've been answering the questions I've posed throughout this book, you're already becoming more aware of your thoughts. However, if you stop at the surface thoughts, the ones you already know, you're not getting the whole picture.

Becoming practiced at not only thought awareness, but going deep enough to pull the whole belief out by the roots is what will help you on those hard days when you don't feel like following through.

I work every day on managing my thoughts. In fact, it's such a habit for me that it's second nature to tap into what I'm thinking most moments of my day. It can be this way for you, too.

This is a practice. I believe it's a very beautiful, soulful practice that can often surprise us. If you're not somewhat caught off guard by what you're thinking, you haven't inquired deeply enough.

Our thoughts aren't always logical or applicable to our lives today. Becoming aware of your thinking for the first time can be like cleaning out an old closet. Not everything in there is useful or even something you remember deciding to keep. There can be old thoughts we picked up from our high school PE class or our first corporate job. There can be thoughts that are completely out of touch with where we are now. We've simply held onto them because we didn't realize they were in there.

You want to make big changes so you can see big payoffs. That is absolutely possible. Learning to practice curiosity about your thoughts is the first step to doing that.

Let's review a list of questions from a previous chapter:

- *What do I think about my weight loss?*
- *What do I think about my MS?*
- *What do I think about my body?*

Write down your answers again (it's okay if they're different than the first time). It helps to write out your answers so you can look at them as opinions. When they're swirling in our heads, we tend to treat them more like law.

For each answer, practice going deeper into what you think. For example, if your answer to the first question on the list above was "I think weight loss is hard," get curious as to why you think that. The answer to why you think it's hard may be, "Because I've tried before and failed." Observe that answer as something you're curious about that's interesting.

If a client said that to me, I would go further by asking, "What does it mean to fail?" Your answer will give you insight into what you think about failure and how that could affect your future success. You may find that you think failing is part of succeeding – and realize that weight loss may not be that hard. On the other hand, you may observe that, to you, failing is proof that losing weight can't be done. Either answer gives much more insight into beliefs and how they play into your actions (or inactions) than the initial, more surface, answer.

Inquire at least four deeper levels for each question on the list, like I've done here. The questions you ask as you go deeper depend on your answers. Get curious and ask questions like you're in a conversation with someone you're getting to know.

Future Focus

When you start getting into the practice of spotting what you're thinking at any given moment, a surge is created that's hard to stop.

And, as with practicing anything, the longer your practice, the better you'll get at doing it.

What you'll get as you become more aware of your thoughts is not only the ability to make changes more deliberately, but leaving certain dynamics, like self-sabotage, by the wayside. You're able to stay the course much longer, and get back on track if you stray. Habits are created more easily and, therefore, certain behaviors become second nature.

What would your future look like if things like working out, not eating if you're not hungry, and staying away from ultra-processed foods were second nature? How would you feel if, instead of having a lot of stops and starts, you had solid years of eating in a way you know your body craves?

When you start recognizing thoughts that stop your productivity, you can move past them more quickly. "I don't know how" becomes "I'll figure it out." "It's not happening fast enough" becomes "It's happening, and here's my evidence." Understanding how your mind works helps you keep that consistency and motivation and, in turn, helps you get better results because you're not starting and stopping.

I used to play a (very bratty) game with myself. I called it the "if I keep doing this, by summer, (or fall, or winter vacation, or the next big event) I'll be skinny" game. I'll give you one guess if I ever won at that game. Until I realized what I was doing, I would torture myself with it because it never panned out. I would then beat myself up about how "I can't do this." Being aware of my deeper thinking ended those games. I realized that I wasn't setting myself up for the future I wanted by pressuring myself. I was creating sabotage and keeping that future far away.

You may still beat yourself up about things (it's human, and I do it, too), but when you've unlocked the mystery of what you're really thinking, you can call your own bluff and stop it whenever you like (whether or not we choose to stop is another question indeed).

Choosing to work with those deeper thoughts is when you see the stops and starts smooth out into consistent constructive action that gets results you want.

Start Where You Are Now

There are a few myths about thinking that need busting.

First, for this process to work you don't have to regress back to your childhood and relive bad memories in order to become more aware of what you're thinking. That can be unnecessarily painful and you don't have to do that for what you're trying to accomplish here.

Second, getting curious about your thoughts doesn't mean you have to understand when you started thinking them in the first place. The only things that matter are that you're thinking them now and whether you truly believe them.

Third, practicing awareness doesn't mean you have to sit and cogitate quietly for hours every day. A common thing I hear is, "I don't have time to understand what I'm thinking." That's like saying, "I don't have time to work on my posture." Do you sit and stand? Then you have time to work on your posture. Do you speak and have feelings? Then you have time to ask yourself what you're thinking that makes you feel or act that way. (You can even do it while you're sitting there, working on your posture.)

Learning how to watch your mind with curiosity and find the real reason you feel upset about not going for that run you promised yourself can provide instant gratification. It'll get you the answer – the real answer. And it may be very different from what you expected.

When you're aware of what you're thinking, you're one step closer to managing your thoughts to support the actions you *want* to take.

You can start by getting curious about what you're thinking. More importantly, you can see very quickly that those first, "obvious" thoughts aren't the whole story. You don't need anything to start this process besides a pen, paper, some questions, and your thoughts.

Ask yourself about the last time you didn't do what you planned, like not sticking to the list at the grocery store. Come to the question with curiosity and simply notice what your answers are. No judgment. There are fascinating thoughts floating around in your head. And, no, there's nothing to be afraid of. They're only thoughts.

There are few things sweeter than identifying a thought that's stopping progress and moving past it to success.

The second you get the hang of that and see results is the second you'll want to do it again.

Chapter 11

Common Pitfalls

B y now I'm sure you know that the process of losing weight and getting healthy for life is not a straight line to done. Let's be honest – if it were, everyone would be well on his or her way. Unfortunately, that's not the case.

There will be ups and downs in your quest to lose weight. There will be times when you're all in and times when you wonder why you bother. There will be times you fail and neglect to get curious about how to do things differently. And there will be times when you take a break from paying so much attention to what you eat, because something else needs all of your attention. There will be times when you're too tired to even think about eating well.

All of those things can and will happen. Not because you're doing it wrong, but because you're human and you're living this thing called life.

A large part of putting a plan together is looking at what is likely to stand in your way. What are the roadblocks? What will tempt you beyond reason or drain your motivation? What will make you want to quit forever? What support do you need (and what will happen if you don't get it)?

All of these questions are imperative to ask. When you start to see the pitfalls of your plan, you can start to move around them. If you do it right, you can even stop them from happening to begin with.

Think about planning to go for a walk. You don't just go out the door and start walking. You think about the weather so that you don't get two steps and turn around because it's raining. You might load a podcast or playlist on your phone so that you don't get bored and end the walk a little early because you start thinking about having *so* much to do that day. It can seem like just regular planning, but look a little closer. You're looking at what can go wrong – like rainy weather or a bored mind, – and you're fixing it before you start.

There are pitfalls with each of the steps presented in this book. Sometimes you only need to know that the pitfall exists in order to avoid it, and sometimes the answer will take more work like I do with the clients in some of the stories I've shared.

With a little work, help, and foresight, all of these pitfalls can be overcome.

While following the steps in this book, here are some of the pitfalls you may encounter:

"I'm really good at first, but then I can't stick to my diet."

When I was dating, I noticed the relationships I was in could be categorized as one of two types: the fast spark or the slow burn. The fast spark connection was great in the first month – we'd have creative dates, go to new places, and have lots of fun together. But those connections would fizzle quickly. Those were connections with (mostly) good guys, but I knew when a relationship started off fast it would end that way, too. Which was fine – because I fell out of interest just as quickly as the person I was dating did.

But then there were the slow burn connections. There were far fewer of those, but they were exclusive and special. Instead of an initial burst of excitement, there was strong mutual fascination and curiosity. We moved along in step as the relationship got more serious. It was beautifully comfortable and yet surprising, and it lasted – you can guess that my husband was in this dating category.

I personally love that burst of motivation and that fast spark of excitement that's full of possibilities. There's crispness to a new routine than can sweep you up along with it.

People get really excited about losing weight and creating a healthy lifestyle. They see the clear benefits and want that result now – like *right now*. They feel like they need to hype themselves up to reach what feels like a huge, but worthy, goal. Maybe there was a health scare or something happened to a friend that gave them a wake up call. And that's great, but what happens quickly is that spark fizzling out.

Think New Year's resolutions. Think new bike. I'm often reminded of that basketball net I begged my parents to get me in the sixth grade. I swore up and down I would use it, only to let it hang there, untouched, after a few days of free-throw practice.

The excitement of newness wears off when there's no real plan in place underneath. Especially when the reason you want a change is because you fear something bad happening, or when there's not a clear picture of the future you want.

The fast spark is a common pitfall when we want to lose weight.

My clients often come to coaching after a few failed cycles of a fast spark (I've had more than a few myself). This initial spark of excitement leads us to bite off way more than we can chew and will almost always lead to burnout. Maybe not for a month or two, but eventually that spark will fizzle. You know you're creating a fast spark when you've switched from lying on your couch to working out five days a week. Or from eating anything you want to choosing a strict diet and making yourself stick with it. Those are not changes that will typically last.

When we're looking for weight loss, we want a nice, slow burn. One that creates a relationship you can stay in, marry, and have kids with. Creating the type of changes you're learning about in this book is no different from creating a good, long-lasting relationship. But this one is the most important relationship you will ever have, because it's with yourself and your body. How do you want that relationship to be? Quick and unsustainable, or lasting and strong?

Do you know when you're creating a fast spark rather than a slow burn as you make changes in your life? Be mindful of your pace, because getting that wrong can set you up for a bumpy ride.

"I second-guess myself a lot."

I've been talking a lot about trusting yourself and making simple, "no-brainer" changes to your food. People can have a lot of trouble as they go through these steps. The biggest resistance comes from letting fear-based decisions take over. Fear-based decisions look like second-guessing yourself and what you're doing. It looks like thinking someone with more "credentials" than you knows more about your body. It looks like trying to change your entire life all at once.

Enacting all of the steps I've outlined in this book may be a big change for you. Relying on yourself for the final word may be scary. I summon my inner rule-breaker to help me with this fear sometimes, and I'm asking you to find that rule-breaker in you. No longer are you a zombie following food trends (trends that often contain foods we know are ultra-processed and unhealthy). Break the rules of the current trends so that you can find what works best for you.

Another fear of this type that I often see is that, upon learning so much about what food and chemicals can do to our bodies, people start to fear food itself. They want to make sure every egg, every chicken, every vegetable they eat is organic, sustainably raised, and gluten-free. I'm a big believer in clean food, and if you stick with this process you will find the specific, healthy foods that work for you. However, there's a big difference between being mindful of what you eat and turning a desire to eat well into a fear of food. The fear will get in your way more than any piece of bread ever will.

"I'm so hungry all I can think about is food."

Feeling a sense of urgency around eating is common. When we're used to eating a diet containing ultra-processed foods that have lots of sodium, sugar and chemicals, our "hunger" is not kind (or clear). Knowing when you're genuinely hungry can be tricky.

When I first started to change my diet, I wasn't doing it in a methodical way. I was following a nutritionist's advice, which still had me eating protein bars and bread – food that I've since realized falls into the ultra-processed food category (even though they were labeled as health foods). I was trying very hard to lose weight through dieting, but still feeding my body the very food that it was desperately trying to tell me was bad for me.

While I was in what I call the "diet fog" (not knowing if what I did was working, but doing it anyway), feeling hungry was like being held hostage. I would try to hold on without eating for as long as I could, and when I finally ate it was with a huge sense of relief. I didn't know at the time that I was setting up a dangerous association with food being a reprieve. What I thought was hunger had absolutely nothing to do with my body needing nutrition. The insecurity I felt when I thought I was hungry was actually my body's withdrawal symptoms as it got rid of food that wasn't healthy for me. But I wouldn't be able to tolerate that dire "hunger" for very long, and so I would often overeat to quell that awful sensation.

You can guess that I didn't keep the weight off that time.

Filling your stomach literally dampens physical feelings in your body, distracting you from what your body is trying to say.

Giving a cupcake to a child to stop their temper tantrum may seem like a good idea. You may think you know why they're throwing a fit, and it may seem like distracting them with a treat solves the problem, but do you really know for sure? Nope. And now you've totally changed the conversation with that child because they have a cupcake and are no longer thinking about their problem. (And now there's a different problem – the hyper child who emerges after eating the cupcake.)

Your conversation with your body is no different. Pains, moodiness, and the urgency to eat aren't hunger; they're your body throwing a temper tantrum. Eating may be a tempting way to stop it. But it's ultimately not helpful.

Remember Jenny from Chapter 4? She was confused about her body's hunger signals because she was disconnected from her body and confusing other sensations with genuine hunger. Sticking with the process of separating genuine hunger from emotions was difficult for her, but as we worked through exploring her hunger she was able to become crystal clear on when she was genuinely hungry and when she just wanted the uncomfortable emotions to go away.

"I don't want to get stuck feeling bad all the time."

One of the biggest roadblocks I see with people learning how to feel their emotions is that they're afraid to feel them.

For you, a roadblock to change may be that you're dismissing emotions by labeling them unhelpful, or deflecting how you feel by changing the subject or busying yourself. But *emotions don't go away until they're felt.* That's why we feel like a ball of anxiety sometimes – that ball is comprised of all the unexpressed emotions that have been packed down inside of us. The fear of them only grows because now they feel like an impending emotional avalanche, and who wants to sort through that mess?

It may sound strange, but positive thinking can turn into a pitfall as well. I believe in positive psychology. I have studied it and taught many classes on its tremendous value. I always use tools with my clients that are rooted in the positive mindset. But anything can be used for wrongdoing – even daisies and unicorns. Trying to stay positive can become another way to avoid emotions that you're afraid to feel.

What you're feeling is already influencing your actions. Trying to ignore how you feel won't make the emotions go away, nor will it change how you're acting. Ignoring your emotions (especially when you're afraid to feel negative ones) will only rob you of the awareness of why you're doing something.

Avoiding emotions can create a nasty cycle. Thinking you don't have enough discipline and needing to get back into gear can create more emotions – such as shame – that you want to distract yourself from by eating. Having a diagnosis of any kind can exacerbate this negative feeling even more.

A plan is definitely needed to break this cycle. The plan I create with my clients is teaching them not only how to feel emotions but also how to know when they're avoiding them.

"My body doesn't really *talk* to me."

We've been living with our bodies forever (in this lifetime, at least). Thinking you and your body already have a strong enough relationship can be tempting. Your body did tell you when you ate bad pad thai that one time. That's good communication, right? Well, technically, yes, but your relationship with your body could be much stronger.

If you had a neighbor who only screamed at you from across the yard when they needed something immediately, would you count them as one of your besties? Probably not. If the only communication you have with your body is when it's screaming at you about an immediate need, you can do much better.

There are a few common pitfalls people run into when they're starting the dialogue with their body that prevents them from having a pivotal relationship. One is that they think the relationship is fine already. Usually because by the time they hear their body, it's shouting, and they're not aware that a calmer connection can exist.

Another pitfall is that they don't hear what their body is saying at all. Silence. But your body is still talking to you, even if you're not listening. A tree falling in a forest still makes a noise, even when no one is there to hear it.

I also see people second-guess the message they get from their body, especially if the message is something they don't want to hear.

The biggest pitfall I see with clients on this issue is thinking their body is numb. This can seem especially challenging if you have actual numbness because of your MS. But the body's message can break through that. Also, numbness is a form of communication.

Thinking there's no wisdom to learn from your body is a big mistake that keeps you disconnected. You won't be able to confidently take control over your own health if you continue believing there's nothing to be heard.

Give your body a chance to speak. Let it know that you're listening – and you may be surprised how quickly it pipes up.

"I would love to work out, but I have too much to do."

I hear a lot of people say that even though they know how beneficial working out is, they still don't do it. If you're feeling resistance to working out, take a look at what you *think* about exercising. When you think of walking, do you picture someone in mom jeans taking a walk in silence? Do you picture people in a gym class working themselves until their limbs feel like jelly? Do you picture exercise that's grueling and boring, like running on a treadmill? Do you picture not being able to get anything done in your day because you have to make time for going to the gym?

People often have these kinds of negative beliefs about exercise. When they picture themselves working out, they see themselves as being bored and miserable while doing it. No wonder more people aren't jumping at the chance to work out.

Another reason resistance comes up is that too much is done right out of the gate. Burnout is real and unnecessary. You can start with a sustainable minimum to do each week. Maybe that's a quarter of a mile walk, three times a week, for example. Something small and doable on even the busiest of days is all you need to do to start. You can always do more when you feel like it.

We make working out way more complicated than it needs to be – often because we hear someone saying we should be doing more, or less, or something different entirely.

Working out to lose weight can create resistance. There's research both ways – that working out won't help you lose weight and that it actually does. Whichever is true, I know that if you only work out because you want to lose weight, it will be hard to stick with it. That's because our bodies release weight when they're ready. There may be weeks when the scale won't move for all sorts of reasons. And if working out hinges on the scale moving, your motivation may take a hit.

When I work with clients, I completely separate working out from losing weight. There are way too many benefits of exercise to stop doing because of frustration about its effect (or non-effect) on weight. I help clients become very clear about why they work out, so that they don't sabotage their workouts when they feel like their weight isn't dropping fast enough.

I always say that starting to work out was one of the best things I've done for myself and my MS. It can be for you, too, if you let it.

"I can't be expected to do this *all* the time."

When we're consistently following a plan, it's fabulous. For me, few things are better than feeling like I'm operating like a well-oiled machine. But what happens when something breaks down? Anything can happen, right? It's called life and sometimes it gets in the way of that perfect consistent record.

Maybe you eat an office donut before lunch. *It's Freddy's birthday. I've been good. A donut won't kill me*, you think to yourself. But then, by lunch, you already have another sugar craving that you may as well satisfy. Next to the donut, another bite of something sweet is a drop in the bucket. By dinner you're in full-on "screw-it" mode. Your day is shot. And the following days aren't as good as you'd hoped they'd be, either. Then you slide into the weekend and, well, you have dinner plans at your favorite restaurant – the one with the bread pudding that's absolutely insanely delicious. Bourbon-soaked raisins? Come *on*.

So, there it is, the anatomy of a failure in dieting. But the pitfall isn't what you might think it is. What derails you isn't the office donut or the made-from-scratch bread pudding. What derails you is missing why you went off the tracks to begin with. There's a reason we do everything, including why we reach for things we know will throw us off track. Especially when that something is sugary and we know eating it will set us up for a week of more sugar cravings.

The pitfall is ignoring *why* you took that donut.

When I coach a client though a "bad" week, we get ultra-curious about what happened. I help them drill down to the moments before they took that bite and go deep into what they thought and how they felt. Quite often clients will be shocked to realize something that hadn't occurred to them at first when they were asking themselves what went wrong. By getting super clear on what they were thinking – and knowing that thoughts are not absolute fact – they are able to build themselves up against the same thing happening again. Or, at the very least, they can cut the amount of time that they stay derailed before they get back on track.

"It's hard to stay motivated when I can't tell if it's working."

If you were to rate your level of motivation on a scale from 1-10, what would it be? If you're like me, your answer would be, "It depends."

Your motivation depends on what you're trying to psych yourself up to do. It depends on how long you've been doing it and how successful you've been at it. It also depends on if you're doing something that was your idea and if your body likes what you're doing.

We talked about all the factors that go into motivation, including giving ourselves credit for what we've done, believing we can do it (not that only someone else can), and actually wanting to make the changes.

But what about factors that take our hard-earned motivation away?

Chances are, there's a mean voice in your head that can take your sense of accomplishment down more than a few notches. We all have this voice in our heads. It's the critical voice that maybe sounds like a mother or a teacher. (Note – it has nothing to do with your actual mother. I'm sure she's lovely. But this voice often sounds like some wise authority figure that you were at one time obedient to.)

This voice is critical of what we do. It doesn't want us to get too big for our britches and so it tries to keep us in check. This voice, which comes from our ego, wants the best for us. It wants us to thrive. But the voice uses scare tactics to get us there, which kills our motivation.

This critical voice tries to push us by withholding validation. It wants us to lose a few more pounds before "real weight loss" is acknowledged. This is the voice that says we're not going down a size; our pants are simply stretching out. This is the voice that says it's only water weight we're losing, and that we have to be 100 percent on point all the time with our eating in order to lose weight. It can be hard to catch this voice in action. If you're like I was, you believe this voice. We all have a version of this voice in our heads, critiquing us pretty much all the time. If you believe what your critical voice is saying and you're talking to someone else who believes his or her critical voice, your motivation will not only take a hit, but you won't even realize that another approach is possible.

Lacking motivation can also become confused with the critical issue of your body saying "no." Sometimes the body saying "no" looks like an utter lack of desire to do something. If that's misconstrued as a simple lack of motivation, we can push ourselves down the wrong path. We can see it as a lack of ability on our part, which will lead to beating ourselves up about all things willpower and discipline.

The truth is, sometimes we're not aware that what our mind decides we should do, our body has already rejected as not good for us.

If we're in tune with why we lack motivation, we can revise our thinking and help ourselves down the right path. Just like with that critical voice, other people you interact with may not have the same type of deep connection that you're forming with your body. So they will push you down that same wrong path and not recognize the subtle ways your body is communicating. Sure, they'll spot it when your body is too tired and has had enough, but they won't be able to spot if your body is telling you that a specific workout or a specific food is at the root of the problem, because they might only see it as a lack of motivation. You're the one who can tell the difference.

The pitfalls that come with motivation can be nuanced and need extra focus to be caught.

"I already know that."

By now you're well versed in Thoughts 101. You have read about being aware of what you're thinking and why it matters. But we're typically not raised to have this awareness. Although I believe 100 percent in the power of managing our minds, I needed to first understand the concept before I embodied the practice in my life.

You may be thinking, *Of course this makes sense.* You may already think that positive thinking has a great power and that we have a role in seeing the glass half empty or half full. But having that basic understanding can be more of a hindrance than a help. I've communicated with people who have a positive thinking quote at the bottom of each email signature, but talking with them gives a very different impression.

Having a basic understanding of a concept and thinking "I already know that" can lead us to believe that we're actually practicing it, even if we're not. That's why really digging into thought awareness is so crucial – because by doing so we can see for ourselves if we're only paying lip service or if we're really implementing that awareness into our lives.

We can also become derailed from the practice of managing our minds because we're not "seeing the proof." There is a space between believing something and seeing it materialize in your world. Just because you work to believe that weight loss is possible doesn't mean you'll wake up 50 pounds skinnier the next day. Our bodies don't work that way. I used to become very discouraged and abandon attending to my thoughts and instead pile on more action when I thought something wasn't working. I know now that piling on more action when my mind isn't supporting what I'm doing is an exercise in futility. When you do that, you're not fixing the root of the problem, you're just prettying up what you see.

Both of these issues amount to glossing over the importance of what you're thinking – by believing you already know it or by believing that actions really are what matter. Either way, you're missing the most crucial part of weight loss: what you think about it to begin with.

Set Yourself Up for Success

With every plan comes a pitfall, and some of them are tough to get past. Some pitfalls need a deeper level of awareness on your part to catch. To complicate things further, if you're getting help from someone, you need to be sure the person you're getting help from has that deeper understanding as well.

When I was first learning these lessons about mind and body awareness, how they fit together and ultimately establish health and happiness, I buried myself in the work. I was fascinated and knew this work was the key to the map of health I couldn't yet make sense of. But solidifying bad habits does not make for a smooth ride.

When I'm in "go" mode, I tend to just put my head down and get it done. From the outside, that can seem awesome and, yes, being this way has its benefits. However, when I tried to lose weight and get lasting, healthy results on my own, it was slow going. Losing weight was possible, but my habit of putting blinders on was ultimately unhelpful, because I was missing so much along the way.

"I've got this" can be a common theme with people living with a chronic illness. We feel like we're on our own and have to look after ourselves. We've been dealt a blow with our illness and can feel like we have to prove something. I personally wanted very badly to prove that I could handle my health and more. I soon realized that "handling it" didn't mean going it alone.

The belief that I had no allies on this path created the ultimate pitfall for me.

If you're going to get help with this problem, it will serve you well to vet who you work with. Make sure they have the same beliefs and understanding as you about what you're working on together. Certainly make sure they have the same connection with their body and can help you with yours. Getting that type of support can make this process go much faster.

The most important thing is to stay the course. That can be really difficult when pitfalls come up. The only way I know how to get around these pitfalls is to have a plan. It can be a pro-active plan for the pitfalls you suspect will crop up, and/or it can be a plan for what you'll do when you're faced with a new pitfall that you didn't see coming.

Asking for help can feel like the ultimate weakness. You're probably sick of asking for help because you feel like you do it too much when it comes to your MS.

I have a lot of clients who feel like they have to prove themselves even as they reach out to ask for help. I'll tell you what I tell them: *you have nothing to prove- you are whole just as you are.*

Your number one goal is to be healthy so you can be there for yourself, and for your loved ones without burdening them. I have the same goal. Watching for all of these pitfalls can set you up for success in obtaining this goal.

Not only now, but for years into your future.

○   ○   ○

What's the fastest way to get over these pitfalls?

Find out by listening to the free downloadable audio.

- What will help me stay on track with my weight loss?
- How do I stop these pitfalls from derailing my progress?
- Will I really be able to see these problems before they happen?

Get answers and get access to a complimentary chat over the phone with me.

Visit **http://www.AndreaHansonCoaching.com/learnmore.**

Chapter 12

Paying It Forward

Y ou've just read about all the steps to losing weight and being healthy well into the future. Some of the most important steps are barely touched on in the world of research and doctors. But they all play an important role in finally finding that combination that works for you.

I'm not saying that research, doctors, and gurus don't have a place at your health team table. They absolutely do. But I hope you have come to realize the importance of you being at the head of that table, filtering all the information you search for through your own filter.

The information in this book is so important because being at your natural weight and having a healthy life not only impacts you as a human, it also impacts your MS. Having a chronic condition unfortunately does not preclude us from being diagnosed with more illnesses. And new illnesses negatively impact our MS by potentially making it more aggressive. I don't know about you, but I would like my MS to stay as docile as possible. Creating truly healthy habits for life is a way to help.

Food in and of itself is complicated. Throw in a bunch of people promising that the answer is plant-based, (or Paleo, or Mediterranean, or high fat and protein) and the issue of what you should eat becomes quite cloudy. There are basics that everyone believes in – what I call the "no-brainer" options – and starting off by eliminating those can give you a huge head start.

If what to eat isn't confusing enough, we have factors like genuine hunger and emotions thrown into the mix. Whether we're hungry or bored can be a crucial question, and how to tell the difference is a skill you can learn how to develop.

The referee in all of these factors regarding weight loss is your body. Your body will tell you when you're out of bounds. It will tell you when you have the ball and are in danger of being booted from the game. This referee is nice and will even tell you when you're playing well.

Your body doesn't lie. And it's the best referee there is when it comes to your health.

You will not get the results you want or the future you envision without making changes that are consistent. You need to be consistent to see results as well as to notice where things need a tweak. Part of making changes for life is that you will always be changing. A consistent practice of supporting your health will make those changes both more apparent and easier to implement. I'm all about making things easier on myself these days (there was a time when that wasn't true).

Your motivation and mindset are your two biggest strategic allies. No action is sustainable if your mind isn't in the right place. If you don't want to do something to begin with, the game is over before it's begun. Motivation is the internal resource that keeps us interested in moving forward. Managing our mindsets makes us sure that we agree with the action we want to make.

The beautiful thing about motivation and our thinking is that they don't depend on anything outside of us.

At the heart of any good plan is the understanding that there will be bumps in the road. Predicting those bumps can give you a head start in planning your route around them. Sometimes, knowing pitfalls exist is enough to avoid them. Other times, you may need a little more help to traverse the gap. But turning away and ignoring pitfalls is what can make you lose your way on this path to lifetime health while living with MS.

I like to think of all the options out there – what diet to chose, how to exercise, what to believe – as a bunch of maps tossed my way. I can look at each map and take a wild guess that it will lead me somewhere beautiful and relaxing, but I don't know for sure by just looking at the patterns of the map. I need something to help me interpret the symbols, so I know if I'm moving toward a landfill or a beach. I need something that shows me whether I'm heading for a cliff or a bullet train station. I need a key to the map.

That key decodes all of the factors having to do with your mind, body and future.

The key to these maps is you. And you're creating it right now through your practice of awareness, attentiveness, and connection with your mind and body.

That key is everything.

Creating a Love Fest

What I love most about having this holistic, long-term approach to weight-loss is that, while you lose weight, you're paying extra attention to your body. This means you're doing double duty. By learning how to communicate with your body and manage your mindset you're also becoming keenly aware of what's normal and what isn't. This skill sets you up for being even more proactive in your MS care. You will become less tolerant to letting issues slide and hyper vigilant in getting them resolved.

This practice that you're learning will create a heightened reverence for your body. This is one of the best things I've gained from practicing these tools.

We each have a guidance system. When I first came to this practice, I felt like my guidance system was broken. You may feel the same way. But we're heartier then we give ourselves credit for. Your guidance system may need some dusting off, but it is still in working condition. And you can strengthen it to all-new levels.

Your guidance system just needs a little love and care.

Some people don't give their body love and care. Some see weight loss as a battle to be fought. Some see having MS as a battle.

For those who have both extra weight and MS, it can be an outright war with their bodies.

But waging war on extra weight and on MS means waging war on yourself. We can't hate ourselves to freedom.

Put down the sabers and breathe deeply. Learning how to lose weight and live well with MS is a collaboration with your body, not a fight against it.

You need that reverence for your body and everything that comes with it in order to understand what it needs to be well.

Fall in love with your body – for life.

Feeling Your Life

Where do you see yourself in 20 years?

What do you want for you and your future?

My guess is that you want to be independent, not having to rely on anyone to take care of you. You probably want the freedom to travel where you want to and to do what you want. You most likely want a naturally thinner body that's maintained without you having to think twice about it. And my guess is you want a career well done and a life well lived.

Think about what a day 20 years in your future will look like. Answer these questions to get specific about that vision:

- *What am I doing?*
- *How do I look?*
- *Who am I with?*
- *How do I feel?*

Take a moment to think about your answers. Get a piece of paper and write a journal entry for a day 20 years in the future. Your writing prompt is to continue writing from: "Today was amazing because..."

First, close your eyes and imagine yourself there. Let yourself feel any emotions that come up when you think about yourself during this day in your future. Soak in how delicious everything feels.

This is your life.

This is possible.

This can be real.

Breaking the Habit

Time will pass, regardless of what you do. You can choose to hang back and do nothing at all. You can choose to keep trusting other people to tell you what to do. Or you can choose to start making deliberate changes in your life that will have you trusting your body and putting yourself in control of your future. Time will continue to pass regardless of the path you choose.

When you start something, a ripple is sent into your future. Why not send a ripple of health? If you've already started practicing the concepts outlined in this book, you're sending ripples into your future. As you continue to practice and to strengthen your health, those ripples will compound on one another to become stronger and stronger.

Nothing you do in life is carried out in a bubble. Everything ripples outward like the water after a stone has been thrown into water. You may have felt like you had no control over where those ripples went, but nothing could be farther from the truth. You can have the ultimate control over how you take care of yourself, how you connect with your body, and how you manage your mind to be in harmony with the changes you want to make in your health.

You've most likely had a habit of deferring decisions about your health. You've relied instead on diets you read in books, or on a study you heard about, or what someone said was "good to do if you have MS."

Every day you work to break the habit of deferring decisions about your health is a day you're talking control of your weight-loss and creating a healthy future with MS.

My Wish for You

My wish is that you now know that having a healthy life while living with MS is possible. Being your natural weight is possible. Having the independent future you crave is possible. I want you to know all the steps to take so that you can secure that future for yourself.

My wish is that you lose weight, feel the healthiest you ever have, and live a happy future.

I want you to understand diet, hunger, and emotions in ways you never thought of before. I hope you get to know how to communicate with your body and your mind, and how to keep your motivation burning. Above all, I want you to know how to keep your health consistent well into your future.

These are all great strategies and will have equally great pitfalls, but my wish is that you will have a plan that helps you navigate around the problems.

It's great to have someone on your side to help you – someone who understands and can help you stay on a plan that is customized for you.

Make this the moment that you start seeing your health differently.

You've surely read books before that inspired you to change and you most likely did – for a while. If you then reverted back to a previous norm, that's okay. That doesn't make you a failure; that makes you a human. I've done that, too.

This time can be different. Above all, commit to changing your health. You can do this on your own, but it will take longer. You can think you're all in on this practice, but you can be only scratching the surface without realizing.

To make this time different, your path has to look like nothing you've done before.

Right now can be the beginning of something new, but it's not a passive process by any means. I hope you take this seriously, get a plan, and do everything in your power to stick with it so that it becomes second nature. Your new plan will become second nature if you work with it.

This new future of yours is something that is absolutely possible.

No more broken promises. No more starting over next week. No more waiting for vacation to be over, or for that knight in shining armor to rescue you. Don't let another year go by trying the same-old and getting frustrated yet again because it doesn't work.

Your weight is nothing to mess around with.

Your MS is nothing to mess around with.

Your future will happen no matter what.

May your future be filled with all that you're dreaming of and more.

      ⊂   ⊂   ⊂

Let's stay in touch.

- Get the free audio and learn precisely what you can do to overcome your weight loss struggle.
- Access more strategies from me on how to lose weight and be healthy for life.
- Talk with me personally, over the phone, to ask questions and get the exact answers to what's next.

Visit **http://www.AndreaHansonCoaching.com/learnmore.**

Acknowledgments

I will be forever grateful for all the support and love I had while writing this book. I never feel like words are enough thanks, but I want to make sure a few people know just how much they had my back along the way.

To Clay – There is no end to the adoration and admiration I have for you. You make me laugh multiple times a day. I am a lucky girl to have such an amazing husband.

To my family – For going through what family does and doing it with grace and honor. I am so proud to belong to this tribe.

To Ruth – For selflessly giving everything – from reality checks to marketing advice. You are a force, and I'm so glad to be walking this road with you. I owe you a lifetime of Tiki drinks.

To Angela – Brace yourself, because I'm going to be really cheesy and say thank you for helping me make my dreams a reality. I knew in grade school that I would write a book. Now I have two.

To the Plumies – I have no other words than you are all truly amazing. I have never before encountered such genuine support and love from a group. I am a stronger person because of your generosity and leadership. I hope I've been able to return a fraction of this goodness back to you.

To Lynne – For providing me with a foundation while I spread my wings. I would not have been able to do this without your support (or your sofa to crash on all these years).

To Brooke – I knew we would work together the moment I was introduced to your work. Call me psychic, but I'm so glad it came true. I am one of the many you have inspired to do their best, go all in, and be proud of the results.

To Kurt – You were one of the first people I turned to for help with my MS. 16 years later, I'm a stronger person for it – literally and figuratively. Thank you for being my friend and my sounding board.

You are all simply the best.

About the Author

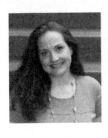

Andrea Wildenthal Hanson is a bestselling author, master certified life coach, and speaker. Since being diagnosed with having multiple sclerosis in 2000, Andrea has learned that the key to living well with MS is being an expert in what works for *you*. Andrea combines her experience from five years of life and weight coaching, and 15-plus years of living with MS, to provide each of her clients with a customized approach to health that includes weight loss and stress management, so that they can live a life they love.

Andrea received a bachelor's degree in psychology from the University of North Texas, and a master's degree in human development, with a specialty in early childhood disorders, from the University of Texas at Dallas. She then became a Certified Life Coach, through Martha Beck, Inc., and became a Certified

Weight Loss Coach and a Master Certified Coach through the Life Coach School.

As well as running her own coaching business, Andrea worked with the National Multiple Sclerosis Society as a coach for their Planning Wise program and for their Every Day Matters program, which focuses on the importance of positive thinking. The Summer 2014 issue of *MS Connections* magazine featured an interview with Andrea about her work with helping people with MS stay employed. She has also run classes for the Memory, Attention and Problem Solving Skills for Persons with MS (MAPSS-MS) research team at the University of Texas at Austin.

Andrea loves green smoothies and recharges her soul by hiking in the mountains. When she's not traveling the world, she lives in Colorado with her husband, Clay, and their perfect dog, Bud Friday.

Thank You

Especially for Readers

Thank you for spending your precious time with me. I hope you enjoyed the book and are practicing first the little nuggets that helped you the most.

Because we've been together for this whole book, I would like to give you a few tools so that you can pack even more of a punch in your weight loss.

First, I have a free audio for you. It's an instant download where I talk about exactly why weight loss when you have MS can seem so hard and I give you direct access to learning precisely what you can do to overcome your weight loss struggle.

*To learn more about the class, visit **AndreaHansonCoaching. com/Learnmore**.*

I also have a customized offer for you. I want to make sure you have everything you need to start down your path of losing weight- for good. I'm offering a complimentary call, so you can ask any questions you like and find out precisely what you need in order to lose weight and have that future you've been dreaming of.

*To schedule, go to **www.callwithandrea.com**.*

These are my gifts to you so you don't have to wonder anymore about what's next. And because who doesn't want a clear path to fast *and* lasting results?

You *can* change your weight.

You *can* change your life.

You *can* change your world.

Here's to losing weight and moving on,

Andrea

A free eBook edition is available with the purchase of this book.

To claim your free eBook edition:

1. Download the Shelfie app.
2. Write your name in upper case in the box.
3. Use the Shelfie app to submit a photo.
4. Download your eBook to any device.

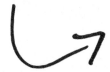

Shelfie

A **free** eBook edition is available
with the purchase of this print book.

CLEARLY PRINT YOUR NAME ABOVE IN UPPER CASE

Instructions to claim your free eBook edition:
1. Download the Shelfie app for Android or iOS
2. Write your name in **UPPER CASE** above
3. Use the Shelfie app to submit a photo
4. Download your eBook to any device

Print & Digital Together Forever.

Snap a photo

Free eBook

Read anywhere

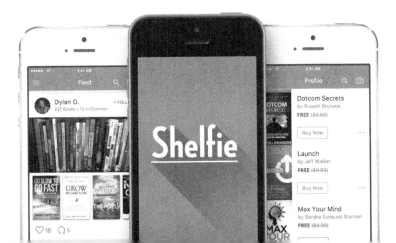

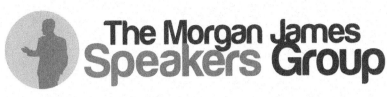

The Morgan James Speakers Group

www.TheMorganJamesSpeakersGroup.com

We connect Morgan James published authors with live and online events and audiences whom will benefit from their expertise.

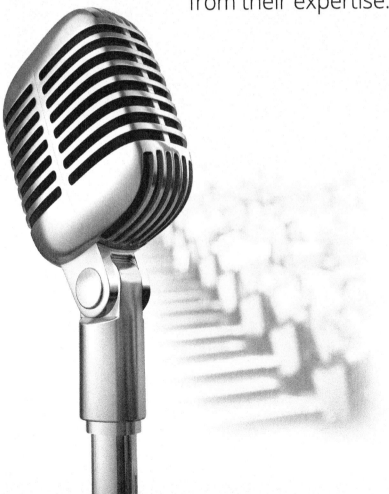

 Morgan James makes all of our titles available
through the Library for All Charity Organizations.

www.LibraryForAll.org

CPSIA information can be obtained
at www.ICGtesting.com
Printed in the USA
BVOW04*1041120517
483970BV00009B/204/P